# PROFESSIONAL
# HAIRSTYLING

GEORGINA FOWLER

NEW HOLLAND

This paperback edition published in 2011

First published in 2007 by New Holland Publishers (UK) Ltd
London • Cape Town • Sydney • Auckland

Garfield House
86-88 Edgware Road
London W2 2EA
United Kingdom
www.newhollandpublishers.com

80 McKenzie Street
Cape Town 8001
South Africa

Unit 1
66 Gibbes Street
Chatswood
NSW 2067
Australia

218 Lake Road
Northcote
Auckland
New Zealand

ISBN 978 1 84773 931 5

Senior Editor **Sarah Goulding**
Designer **Lisa Tai**
Photographer **Paul West**
Production **Marion Storz**
Editorial Direction **Rosemary WIlkinson**

10 9 8 7 6 5 4 3 2 1

Reproduction by Pica Digital Pte Ltd, Singapore
Printed and bound by Craft Print International Ltd, Singapore

# contents

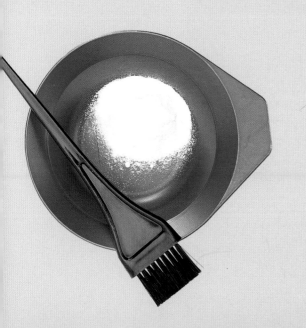

# introduction

The purpose of this book is to prepare you for working in the hairdressing industry and to help develop your skills by providing essential knowledge in all areas of hairdressing. It guides you through easy to understand sections about the different skills you need, with straightforward step-by-step instructions and photographs.

**The book starts with the philosophy of hairdressing** – a look at the hairdresser's world and how we are often perceived by others, the hard work, the competition and the importance of customer service. By facing the facts, it will help to build your confidence and prepare you for the hardworking world of hairdressing.

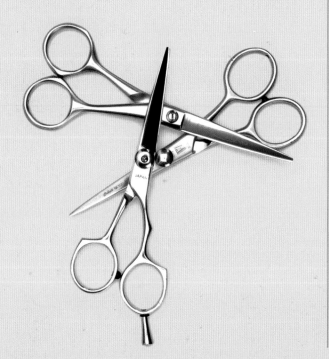

**The Tools section** looks at some of the essential items which are needed to deliver hairdressing to a good standard, with explanations of how and when to use them. The tools and equipment that a hairdresser might need could fill a book by themselves, but I have listed some of the more important items that a hairstylist may need on a day-to-day basis. The tools section also includes tips and some trade secrets that will give you some extra guidance.

**Getting the Right Results** focuses on the importance of consultation. This will help you to maximize the information you can get regarding a client and their hair, directing you through how to consult and the questions to ask. This should help you to obtain the perfect end results that a client will be pleased with.

**Down to the Roots** covers the four main sections of hairdressing: shampooing, cutting, colouring and perming. These form the backbone of hairstyling, and are vital skills to master. First we cover simple techniques to guide you through a perfect shampoo, then cover how to apply

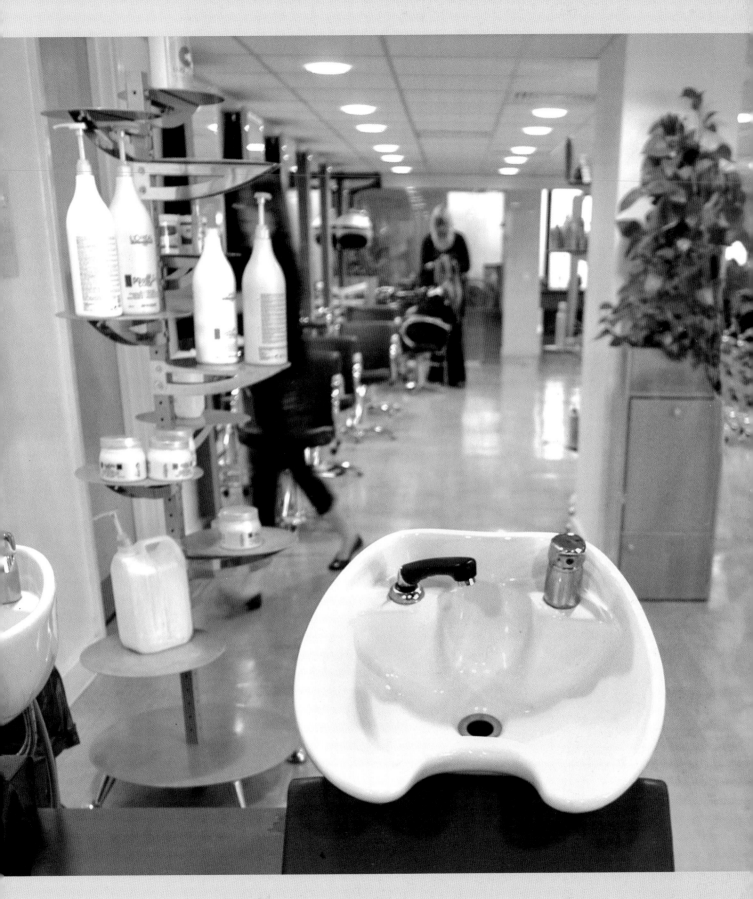

conditioners and treatments correctly. This section also includes head massage techniques to treat your clients to.

Step-by-step photographs and text take you through four basic cutting techniques, with a fifth section on personalizing cuts using techniques such as slicing, thinning and giving texture to hair. From this you will be able to recreate the looks on anybody's hair.

The section on colouring hair looks at hair chemistry and goes back to basics with how colours are made up, the pigments in natural hair and how to diagnose them, and gives you an insight into all the hair colouring products

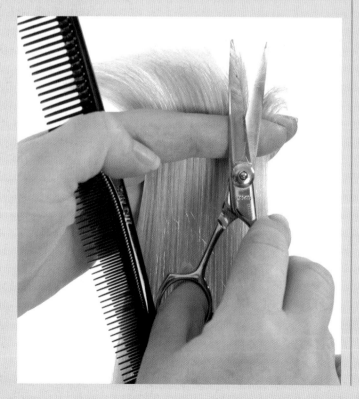

available on the market, how long they last and why. Step-by-step instructions and photographs will help you to apply the colours perfectly. The actual selection of colour is also very important. We'll help you to make it easy to achieve great results that keep your clients happy, with tips and trade secrets and finally a guide on some new and exciting applications for different colouring looks, which can be used on either men's or women's hair.

Even though perming is gradually falling out of favour, it is still vital for any hairdresser to understand the chemical process and know how to do it. The perming guide will equip you with all the latest knowledge on this application, teaching you about the structural build of the hair bonds and how perming on the hair works. It also instructs you on what wind technique to use and why, which lotions to use, and gives you pointers on how to deal with the aftercare, correcting any problems and what advice to give to a client.

**The Male** looks at men's hair cuts – also a big part of the hairdressing world. This short section on men's hairstyling should help to give you inspiration and guidance on cutting men's hair, including a step-by-step guide on short cut clipper work and why cutting men's hair is really no different to cutting women's.

**Formal Invite** has easy to follow instructions that will enable you to create three perfect looks for a client to attend a special event. Whether it's for a wedding or a cocktail party, we will take you through putting up hair and the accessories and equipment needed to finish an elegant look for any occasion.

**Salon Genius** offers some helpful pointers on how to start your own business, make money and maximize the potential. Some guidelines to help you find the right premises and on the look you want to create for it should also help, along with notes on customer service, dealing with complaints and different ways of getting started.

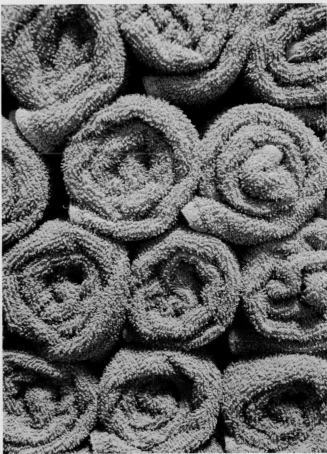

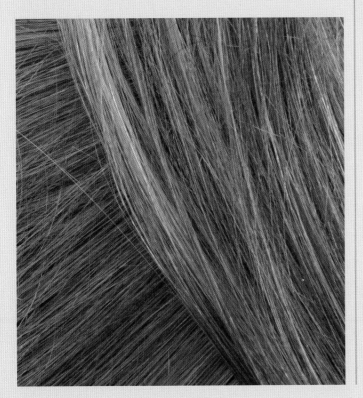

**Business Checklist** follows on from this, and looks at the different businesses you can become involved with, how to finance them, your legal obligations and costs, staffing, equipment, and finding the perfect location. Top tips and great advice should give you the headstart you need to succeed in the competitive world of hairstyling.

All of the essential information in this book should help you on your way to becoming a hairdresser with great potential. With plenty of practice and the help of this book, you can acquire great basic knowledge and skills and some firm foundations for your hairdressing career.

# the philosophy

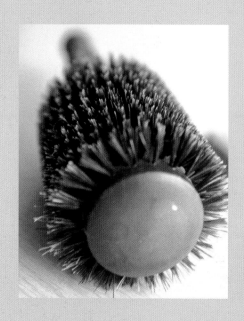

Over the years I have heard all the jokes – that hairdressers don't know the meaning of hard work, that we sit around talking all day about the weather and holidays and drinking coffee. The reality is quite the opposite – a lot of people don't see the real hard work that is required, standing for most of the day and often having very short lunch breaks, having to eat quickly or in between clients.

You will find that many people think hairdressers are unintelligent, but you will soon realize that hairdressing is not only a highly-trained skill, but a profession, as well. It might only take two to three years to become fully qualified, but it takes many years of experience to become a real professional. In this sense it is a little like learning to drive – qualifying doesn't take long, but the more practice you get, the better you become and, in the case of hairdressing, the better your reputation will be. Hairdressing might not require the same intelligence as for becoming a doctor or a lawyer, but it is still a profession that requires skills in maths, science, language, communication skills and art, not to mention common sense.

If you are thinking about a career in hairdressing, be warned that the hours are often long and the pay is not brilliant to start with. Having said that, however, the rewards increase as you progress if you own a business or are just really great at what you do, as people will pay a lot of money for good hairstyling. Tips can be an excellent bonus of the job and are common, and the majority of managers offer commission incentives to their staff. These can earn you good money, although you have to work hard for it.

Perhaps the hardest part of hairdressing is the customer service. Dealing with the public in most jobs is demanding, but physically changing the way someone looks is particularly risky. It is also surprisingly hard to talk to people all day; people with whom you often have nothing in common. The reason hairdressers often talk about the weather or holidays is not because they are dull – it's just sometimes the easiest way to open up a conversation with someone you know nothing about. And it works – people tell you all sorts of things when they are comfortable with you, and you can often lend a sympathetic ear as part of the service.

You are constantly being educated in hairdressing, and gaining a qualification alone is not enough. Styles, fashions and techniques change rapidly, with new technology and new ways to cut or do technical things such as colouring. It is vital, therefore, to keep educating yourself with new courses and product knowledge.

In summary, hairdressing can be as exciting or as boring as you make it. If you're motivated and inspired you will learn much and go far, and can earn a good living from it. If you just want to plod along then that's fine too, if less rewarding. The huge advantage of a skill such as hairdressing is that it goes with you anywhere you go, and is a skill that requires very little but a pair of scissors and a comb as the bare essentials.

Georgina Fowler

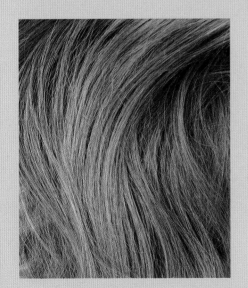

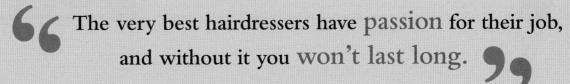

**The very best hairdressers have passion for their job, and without it you won't last long.**

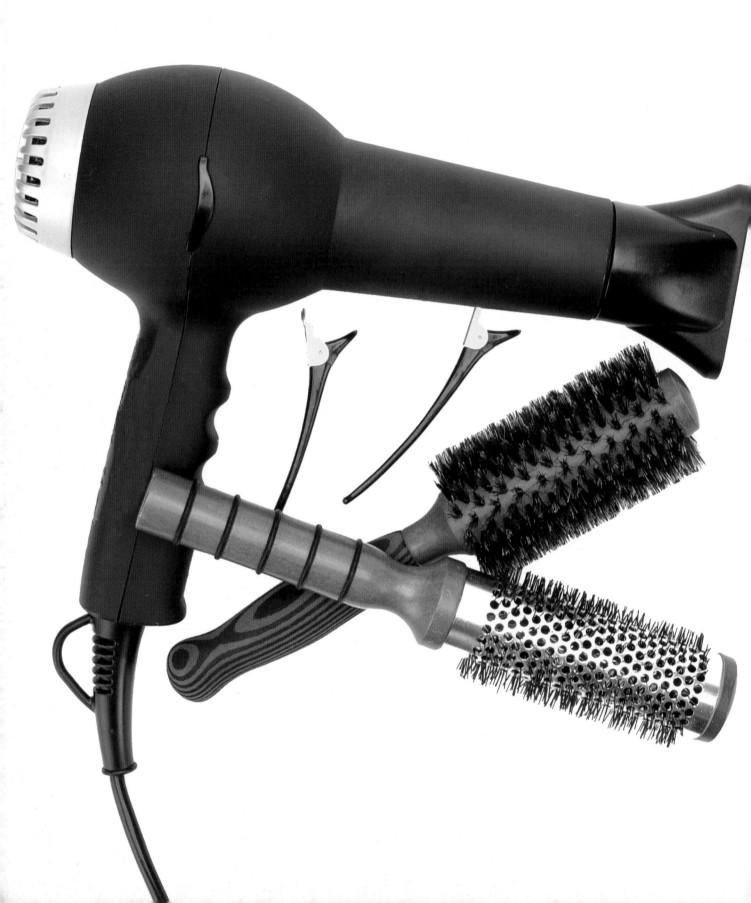

# 01 the tools

# combs

In hairdressing, combs and brushes are essential tools of the trade. Without them it's almost impossible to create some of the looks we illustrate in this book. Combs range hugely in size, shape and the material in which they are made. Below are a selection of combs available, but certainly not the only combs you will see in the industry.

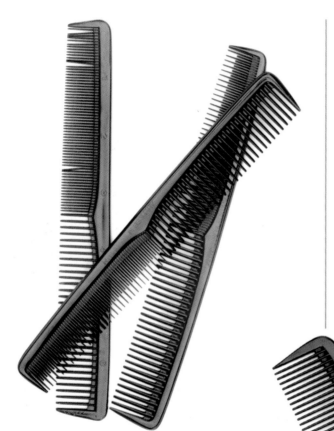

## Tail comb

A tail comb is used mainly for colouring, perming, setting and putting up hair, as the prong is useful for separating and weaving out strands or sections of hair. The other end is like a regular comb and is used for combing knots out of the weaved or separated strands. When used for setting, a tail comb is good for taking sections of hair.

Tail combs vary in size and the material they are made of. There are both plastic-ended and metal-ended tail combs – personally I prefer the metal-ended type, as a plastic-ended tail is often too thick to take a fine weave. It is also much wider than the fine end of a metal-ended tail comb.

## Cutting comb

Used mainly for cutting and sometimes for combing out wet hair, cutting combs often have two different rows of teeth from one end to the other. One end has finer, closer teeth; the other has slightly wider-set teeth for thicker hair. The comb is also often wider at one end and thinner at the other. The actual comb size also varies, which is for the comfort of the person using it. Be aware that some cheaper combs can be made of cheaper material, so can bend when combing thicker hair, or even snap, as they are not strong.

## Wide-tooth comb

A wide array of combs fit into this category, but generally they are good for use prior to cutting or when the hair is wet, perhaps with conditioner on. As the name suggests, wide-tooth means that the teeth are set wide apart, so enabling you to comb out knots and snags from the hair easily. Again, this comb comes in many shapes and sizes.

# brushes

Brushes also come in all shapes, sizes and materials. It is worth investing in a variety, as all of them will come in useful at some point in your hairdressing career.

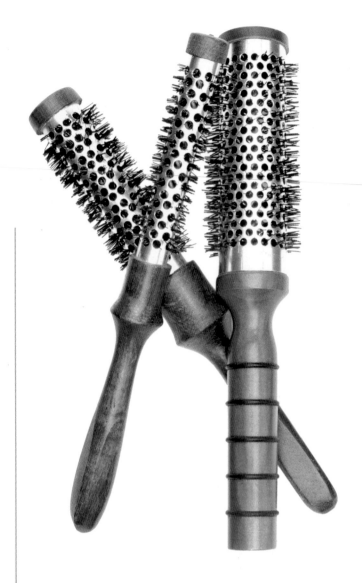

## Circular brushes

There are a great many different sizes of circular brush, from the smallest round brush the size of a packet of sweets, to very large round brushes with the circumference of a mug. The barrel of a circular brush comes in several different materials, the two most common being metal and nylon. The main difference between the two is that the metal barrel heats up when you dry with it, so it helps to set the hair into place rather better. However, a nylon or wooden barrel is a lot softer on long hair and can be left in the hair like a roller while you carry on blow-drying the next section with another brush.

Circular brushes are used on all lengths of hair, and it does not necessarily follow that you have to use the smallest one on short hair – small circular brushes can be good to get into the roots of long, curly hair when a client wants you to dry their hair straight.

## Denman and vent brushes

Denman brushes don't seem to be used as much these days, but if you ever need to do a set, they are good for brushing out the heavy set curls that leave lines in a client's scalp. They are now more commonly used by non-professionals as an everyday brush, but they are still great brushes for dressing out hair that has been blow dried.

A vent brush has very wide-spread prongs with gaps in between them, and is always made of a heavy, strong plastic. It is a very good hair-drying brush. By contrast, a

Denman brush has a solid rubber spine which the more condensed prongs come through. The prongs are a lot closer together, which makes it a lot stronger for brushing out hair.

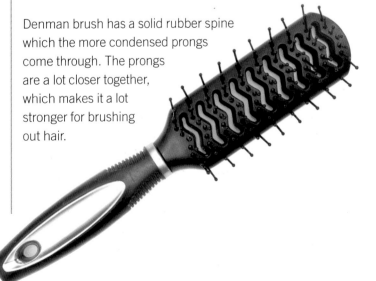

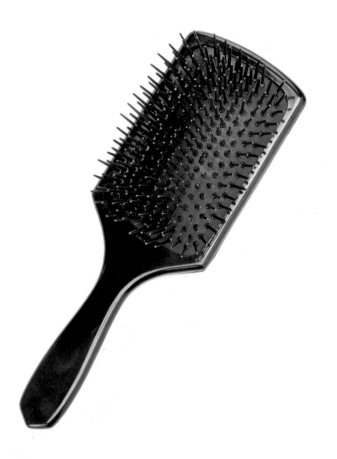

## SNAPPER BRUSH

Snapper brushes have become very popular recently, and look like two flat brushes or paddle brushes facing each other and attached at one end. They are easy to control and look much like straightening irons with bristles – and are used in much the same way. To use, you 'snap' a section of hair at the root inside the brush, put your blow-dryer on it and pull it down the hair to the end. The bristles of the brushes are cut very short – if they were too long, the brush would not snap together as well.

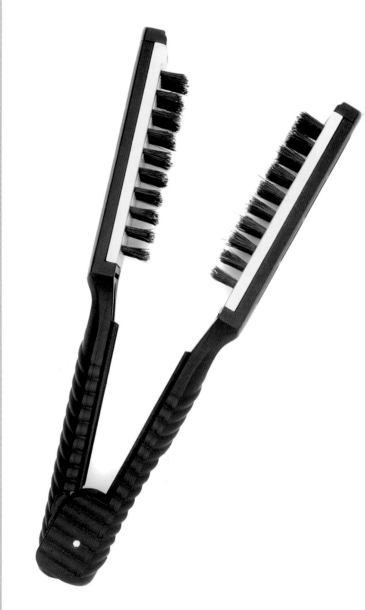

## PADDLE BRUSHES

Paddle brushes have been used for hundreds of years and have recently become popular again. They are made by many different companies and come in many sizes, but they are generally flat, hence the name. They are quite soft to the touch, as often their bristles are made of a softer material. They are mostly used for helping to dry hair straight, as they are easier for someone to use themselves, as opposed to using a circular brush which can get tangled up in your hair. They may take a while to get used to, however, as they are not used like most brushes which are twisted around whilst drying.

## SOFT BRUSHES

These brushes are excellent when doing put-ups or dressing hair after back-combing. They smooth over the top of hair and don't brush right down to the scalp if used correctly. They come in many shapes and sizes, but often the bristles are very soft and flexible, bending and moving slightly.

# dryers and attachments

Along with scissors, hairdryers and attachments are a vital tool of the trade, especially with the old hood dryers disappearing quickly. Having the right dryer and attachments can make a huge difference to your finished look.

## Hairdryers

Hairdryers have come on in leaps and bounds since they were first invented, when they were large, unwieldy contraptions made of metal and wood. These days we have super-light versions with any number of speed and power settings: ultra light turbo, super turbo, 1,600 watts, 1,800 watts and even 2,100 watts, boosting the power you have and the speed at which the hair dries. They come in many different colours, makes and every shape and size to suit the user.

There is a difference between professional dryers and regular dryers. It used to be the shape, as you could always tell a professional dryer from its long neck, whereas regular hairdryers were short and stubby. Now even the regular dryers have followed suit, but they don't have the same power. Check the wattage, which will tell you how strong it is – professional dryers are usually 1,800 watts and above.

Professional hairdryers just used personally at home will last for many years, but of course in a salon using them day in and day out, blow-dry after blow-dry, you will find that the lifespan is not as long. From my personal experience I would say that they last about one to two years before they burn out.

To prolong a hairdryer's life, it helps if you clean the filter regularly and try not to drop it too often! Also have the wiring checked every now and again – in a salon, the salon owner should by law have all electrical equipment tested regularly, at least once a year.

## Attachments

### NOZZLES

Most professional stylists like to use a nozzle on their dryer. Some don't, and the choice is yours, but bear in mind that with a nozzle you can direct the air from the dryer into certain places on a brush or on to hair for more precise drying.

### DIFFUSERS

This is a large, circular disk that attaches to the end of the hairdryer. It softens the airflow, so when directed at the hair it does not blow it everywhere. It is mainly used for curly hair, as it allows the curl to dry almost naturally.

# heated equipment

Heated appliances are extremely popular these days, particularly straighteners and curling tongs, depending on whether the fashion is for poker-straight hair or soft waves. There are also other heated tools that will finish a style after blow-drying.

## Heated rollers

Often used after a blow-dry or before a put-up, heated rollers help to boost the hair's volume and give bouncy curl. They are normally purchased in a box that heats up by plugging into the mains. The rollers stand on rows of metal sticks and heat from the inside out. Some more expensive brands have a temperature gauge and will automatically light up when ready to use; more old-fashioned rollers have a little dot on the top that changes colour when hot.

The rollers are pinned into the hair with a special pin-type prong that slides over the roller to hold it in place. Some versions have different clips to hold them, such as snapper clips.

As with all heated equipment, treat with caution and make sure the wiring is tested on a regular basis.

## Straightening irons

Straighteners have enjoyed a surge of popularity in recent years, and they are used extensively both in salons and in homes. Don't allow their popularity to prevent you from learning how to dry hair correctly, however – it is still vital for a professional to learn this skill.

To use, slide them down the already blow-dried hair from root to tip – you are essentially ironing the hair with intense heat.

Always remember that straighteners can heat up to very high temperatures and can be dangerous if left unattended. Make sure that they are tested regularly and always turn them off after use.

## Tongs

These are a similar tool to the straightening irons but create curl instead of straightness. They are used for many things, from finishing short blow-dries to curling lengths of long hair into spirals, or even to finish a put-up. They can can get extremely hot and need to be used with care.

To use, take a small section of hair and put the end of the hair in between the snapping piece of metal and the tong itself. Wind the hair around the tong until just close enough to the scalp without burning and leave for a few seconds before unwinding. A good tip is to slide a comb under the tong, in between the tong and the scalp, in order to prevent you from burning the head.

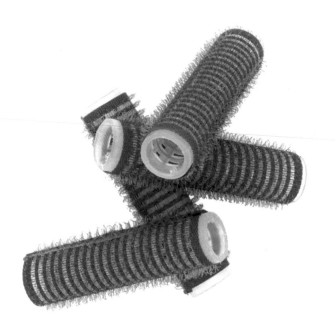

## SETTING ROLLERS

These old-fashioned rollers are plastic and come in different sizes and colours to match. They have small gaps in between the grids of the roller through which you slide a plastic pin, to hold the roller close to the head. Generally these are used for wet sets and have been around for many years.

When setting with these rollers, you would generally section the hair into small sections and pin each individual roller into place. They are then secured with a hair net to stop them falling out and ear foams are provided – hood dryers have a tendency to get too hot and burn the ears.

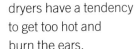

# Rollers

## VELCRO ROLLERS

These rollers stick very easily to the hair on their own, with no clips required. They come in different sizes and are coloured according to size. The main drawback with Velcro rollers is that they don't make a clean, crisp curl, as when removed they tend to pull odd strands of hair with the roller. However, they are very quick and easy to use, and they are versatile – they can be used on wet or dry hair and can be put in day-old hair to help revamp it.

## BENDY ROLLERS

Bendy rollers were originally used for perming, but they have gradually made their way into the setting world for both professionals and non-professionals. They can be rolled into dry or wet hair to create softer waves that have an 's'-bend look to them. They have a metal inner that allows them to bend into shape, and a sponge outer shield to protect the hair. They come in several different sizes which are normally represented by different colours. To get better results, use an end paper to make sure the ends are tucked in properly.

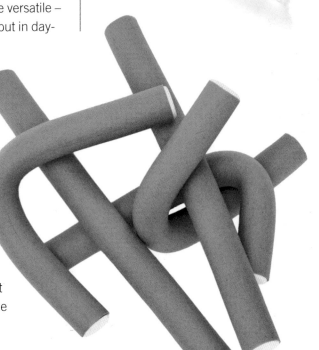

# styling products

There is a vast array of styling products now on the market made by many different manufacturers, but generally speaking many of them are similar products bar the branding. What follows is a rough guide to what each product is and what they are used for.

## Mousse

Used as a styling aid prior to blow-drying or setting on wet hair. Usually creates volume and body and can come in colours, too, to enhance. Ranges in strength of hold from soft to extra firm.

## Volume spray

Used as a styling aid prior to blow-drying or setting on wet hair. Used mainly for volume and for giving lift to the roots area of hair. Normally comes in one strength. Avoid using too much, or the hair will be weighed down.

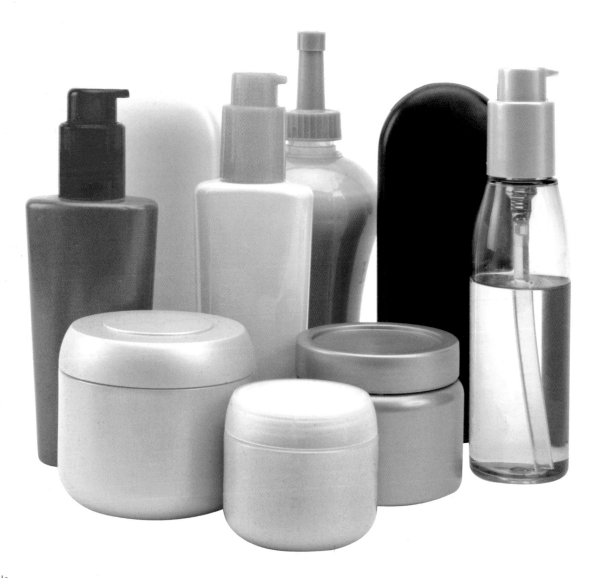

## Thermal spray

Used with heated equipment such as tongs, straightening irons or heated rollers to help protect the hair from heat damage. Can sometimes come in different hold strengths.

## Thermal cream

Often used with heated styling equipment – normally straighteners – as the cream helps to put lots of moisture in the hair and also keeps the hair smooth. This protects the hair from heat damage.

## Straightening cream

Can come in gel, cream or serum form, and is used as a styling aid prior to blow-drying to help smooth and straighten the hair. It doesn't usually have a hold strength as it is more for softening and smoothing.

## Curl enhancers

These come in sprays, gels or creams and are used as a styling aid prior to blow-drying or natural drying to help isolate and enhance curl in the hair. The product sometimes has a light hold.

## Thickeners

Used before drying on wet hair and help to give thickness and body to it. Can come in different hold strengths, though some may have no hold at all.

## Serums

Often used prior to or after a blow-dry or set to help smooth frizzy or dry ends. They can seal split ends, and can sometimes help to make hair straight. Often an oil-based product, so you need to be light on use if hair is fine as it can get a little oily.

## Wax

Used as a finishing product to style and mould hair into shape. Can also be used on the ends of long hair to define a look, and available in various different strengths.

## Gel

Used as a finishing product. Can give a 'wet look', but can be used on both wet and dry

hair. Comes in a range of strengths, but firm hold is common. Works very well on short styles.

## Pastes/pomades/clays/muds

So many new and exciting styling and finishing products are now available that it's hard to keep up, but generally these sort of products have different holds and textures for different looks and lengths of hair. Experiment with as many as possible to get a better idea of what each one does.

## Shine sprays

Used purely for generating shine on a finished style.

## Hairspray

Used to hold a finished style in shape. Sometimes hairsprays can be a wet spray and in pump-action bottles these take a minute or so to set. Most are still in an aerosol form and come out as a fine mist. The strength of the hairspray depends on the type.

There are so many styling products on the market now that this is not an exhaustive list. It is a good idea to try and test as many different products as possible – you may find a range you prefer from one company, or you may like to mix and match products from lots of companies.

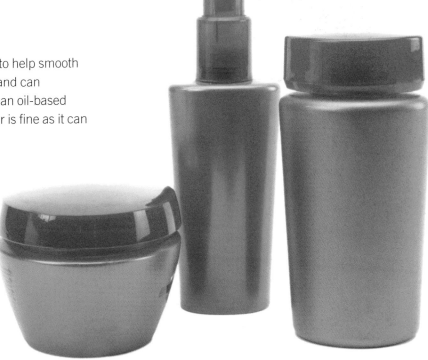

# miscellaneous tools

There is a wealth of miscellaneous equipment that is needed for hairdressing. These tools are often left out of pre-prepared kit bags, but they play an important role in the life of a stylist. Make sure you have at least some of the following.

## PPE: personal protective equipment

By law, there is equipment that should be used and supplied during certain work in the hairdressing industry. Just like a builder has to wear a hard hat, a hairdresser must protect themselves from injury or damage. Protective items include:

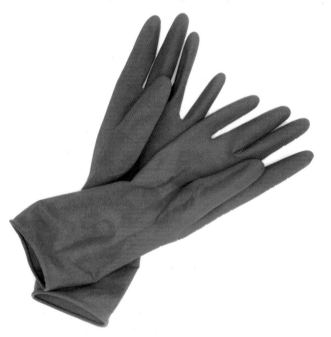

**Gloves** – You can either buy gloves that are reusable or disposable gloves. These protect hairdressers' hands from chemicals such as colouring products, bleaches, perm lotions and chemical relaxers. Without protection there is a chance of contracting dermatitis which, if severe, can prevent you from continuing hairdressing as a career.

**Aprons** – It is wise to use these during colouring, perming and relaxing processes. They protect your clothes from spillages and can prevent damage. It is also advisable to cover your client with a cape of some sort, as they also need to have their clothes protected from any possible spillages or damage.

## Miscellaneous equipment

There are many miscellaneous items in hairdressing. Below are some of the most common that you will need.

**Clips** to pin hair out of the way during cutting or colouring.

**Bowls** to mix colour in or put neutralizer in for perms.

**Measuring jugs** to measure out colours and oxidants.

**End papers** for perms.

**Sponges** for applications of colour or neutralizer.

**Foils** for colouring.

**Cotton wool** for removing excess colour or for protection from perming.

**Hair bands** or elastics.

**Hair nets** for put-ups.

**Clingfilm** which can be used to wrap the head with and retain heat for colouring.

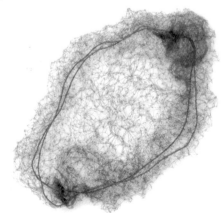

# trade secrets and tips

## TO IMPROVE YOUR HAIRDRESSING

- Don't overdry. When you blow-dry, make sure that the hair is almost, but not completely, dry. Leave some moisture in to prevent static.

- When blow-drying curly hair straight, use a small, round brush at the roots. A big, flat brush or large, round brush will not get right into the roots with the heat of the dryer, which prevents it from straightening properly.

- When shampooing oily hair use tepid water and do not scrub, which most people want to do as they feel it cleans their hair better. It actually stimulates the sebaceous glands to produce more oil. Tepid water helps to stop stimulation, whereas hot water will add to the problem.

- If the hair always lies flat due to a crown or double crown, using the correct styling tools and drying the problem area in the opposite direction (to redirect the hair and give it more lift) will help. Don't dry the hair flat to the head, as it magnifies the flatness in the crown area. Instead, use a brush to lift the hair off the scalp. If the hair is sticking up in the crown area and you have short hair, try growing the hair longer. You should find that the weight of the hair will cover and disguise the crown.

- To help straighten out a cowlick (a swirl of unruly hair that won't comb down properly), dry the hair from wet, forward over the forehead with a round brush or small paddle brush and use a product of some sort. This will weigh down the cowlick, making it easier to put into style.

- To limit drying out or damaging the hair when using heated styling equipment such as straighteners, tongs or heated rollers, use a thermal protective product. This will not make the hair sticky or solid like a setting spray, but will protect the hair from the excessive heat.

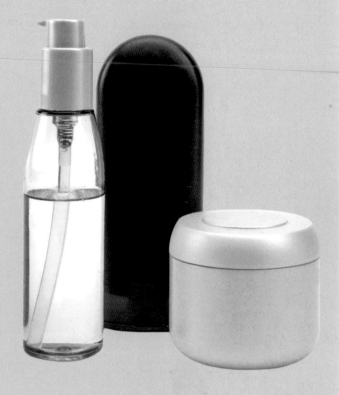

- Leave-in conditioners are perfect for the beach, as they generally contain sunscreens to protect hair from sun damage.

- When using hot rollers, spray dry hair first with a fine hairspray. Take your first section and comb it smooth, spray with hairspray and then twist the section before wrapping it on the roller. This will give a spiral look to the curls. After the rollers have cooled, take them out and spray with a fixing hairspray. Finally turn the head upside down and run your fingers through the hair.

- To get super straight hair without frizzing, always use the nozzle on your hairdryer and aim it downwards. Hold the hair straight as you are blowing it dry, and use cool air to finish. This will set the shape.

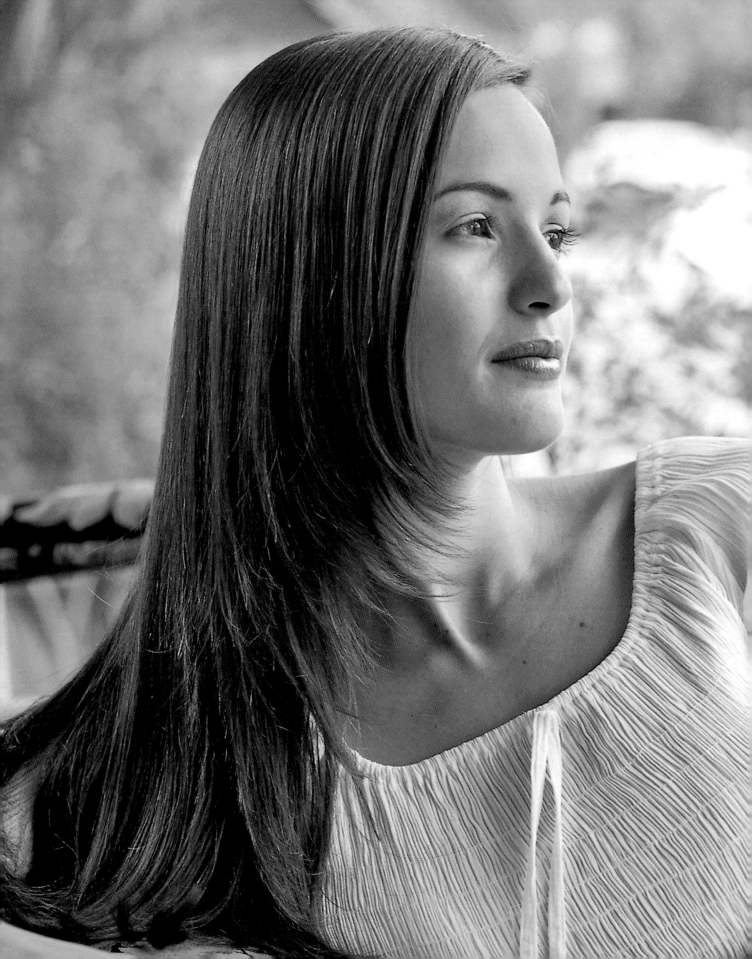

# 02 getting the right results

# consultation

When a client comes into a salon to get their hair done, one of the most important parts of the whole process is the consultation. This should never be overlooked – it really does not matter how good you are at cutting, colouring or perming; without a full and detailed consultation, even the best hairdresser will fail to get the best result. A consultation gives you valuable information to help you deliver the perfect hair.

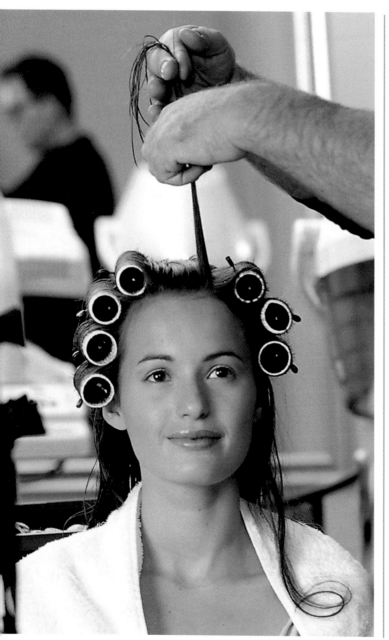

## Face shape

When looking at potential styles, the first thing you should do is identify the client's face shape. When you are first trained you will do this very deliberately, but once you have become more qualified you will find that, although you do look at the hair and face shape, you will do it almost unconsciously and will be better at knowing instinctively what hairstyle would be best.

Faces come in many shapes and sizes, all of which can alter the way a hairstyle turns out. Identifying which face shape you are dealing with can help determine where the hair would lie best and the how thick it should be in certain areas. An oval face is the easiest shape to work with, as it will suit almost any cut. Not many of us have the good fortune to have this, however, so what a hairdresser does is to work with what they have, creating a look that tricks the eye into thinking a face is oval.

It is very important to remember, however, that this is one of the many areas in hairdressing where, ultimately, the customer is always right. You may have a hairstyle in mind that you think would suit the client much better, but if they are comfortable and happy with a style that you perhaps feel isn't suited to them, it does not mean you should necessarily change it. Offer advice and make suggestions by all means, but if they are resistant to your ideas or keen to try a different style, you must respect their wishes, whatever your personal opinion might be.

To find out what your own face shape is, pull all your hair back from your face and look straight-on into a mirror. Trace the outline of your face onto the mirror – this should give you a general idea of your face shape, although bear in mind that side and three-quarter profiles are also important when deciding on a hairstyle.

## DIFFERENT FACE SHAPES

The 'perfect' face shape from a hairstyling point of view is oval, and stylists often try to create the illusion of an oval face by cutting the hair accordingly. For example, a long face face does not need to be elongated by long hair – it is best with shorter hair and some type of fringe to soften the length of the face. A triangular 'A'-shape would need more hair up top, preferably with some weight to fill out the top of the 'A', but would not need more hair around the jaw area as this is already quite broad.

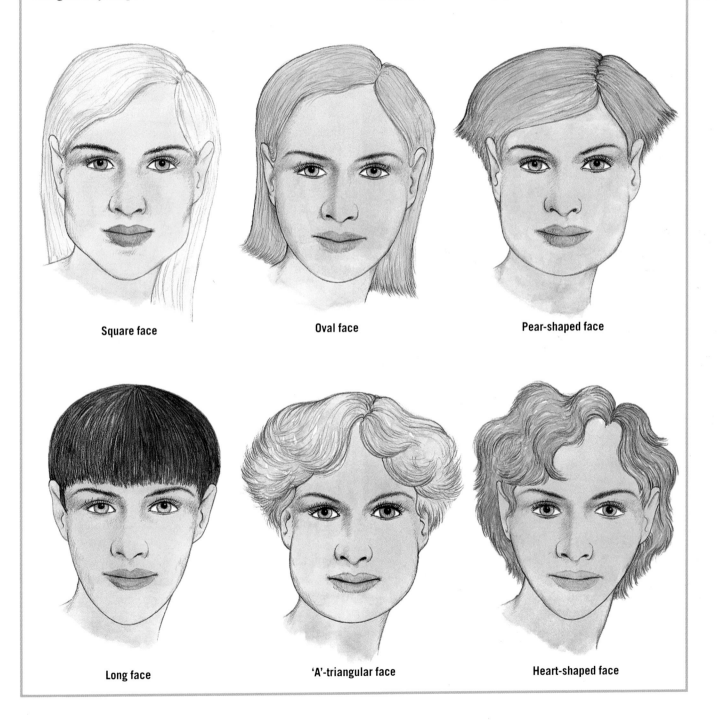

**Square face**

**Oval face**

**Pear-shaped face**

**Long face**

**'A'-triangular face**

**Heart-shaped face**

# asking the right questions

It is important to establish a good relationship between yourself and the client when consulting. Not only will this get the best results, but it makes your job more pleasant and makes it more likely that the client will return to you in the future.

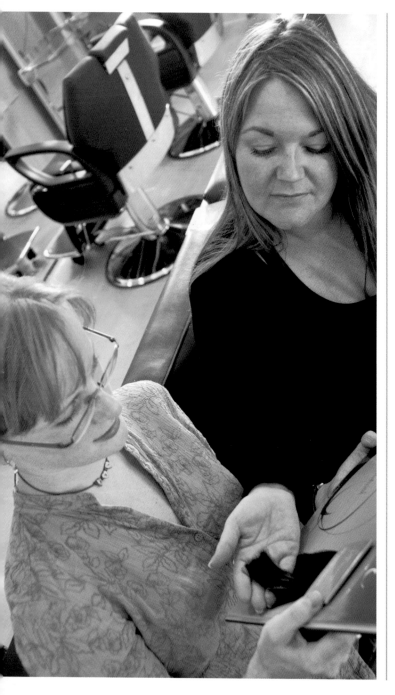

Consulation should always be done using open-ended questioning techniques, specifically what, where, when and how. For example, 'How often do you have your hair cut?'. The answer to this could be anything from sometimes, rarely, every 8–12 weeks or every 6–8 weeks. Closed questions, such as 'Do you cut your hair every six weeks?' will elicit only a yes or no answer and will make life harder for you. Open questions often lead to a natural conversation and will give you much more information.

## ZONES

Using the right 'zones' when dealing with a client is very important. Zones indicate how close you should be to a client when talking to them, and there are three basic zones:

1 = unfriendly, cold – too much distance between you and the client.

2 = comfort – just the right distance so as to be close but not too close.

3 = uneasy – too close and in the client's face.

The second zone is obviously the one to aim for and will be the most comfortable for both you and the client.

Understanding body language is a great skill to master as a hairdresser. It can tell you a lot about the mood of a person, so look out for telltale signs especially when you have finished the hair, as it will tell you if your client likes what you have done.

A good ice-breaker for when a client first meets you is for you to put your hand lightly on their arm, welcome them and then introduce yourself. Most clients can tell how confident

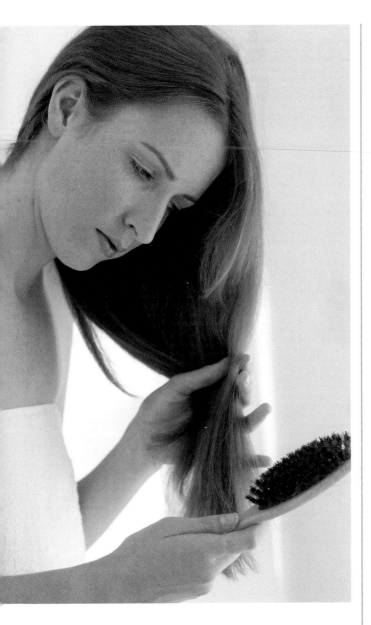

## Tests

There are some tests that you are strongly advised to perform on a client's hair prior to any chemical treatments, and also some tests to perform prior to cutting and styling. They may also help when advising clients on which products to use.

### POROSITY

Running your thumb and forefinger from the roots to the ends of a few strands of hair will show how porous the hair is. If it seems to have a ridged feeling and is bumpy as you move your fingers down the hair, it means it is porous; if it is smooth, it is normal. This will help you to judge how well the hair will take colour.

### ELASTICITY

This is best done when the hair is wet. Take a few strands of hair and lightly stretch them like pulling an elastic band. If the elasticity is good, the hair should only stretch a tiny amount that you can barely feel or see. If the elasticity is poor, it will stretch like an elastic band and will not return – it will break and possibly snap off. This is poor elasticity and tells you that the hair is very fragile. Treatments for reconstruction would be a good idea at this point and very little else – not even blow-drying, as this also weakens the hair.

### SKIN TEST

This should be done when planning any colouring, and should be done at least 24 hours in advance to make sure that there are no reactions. It is done by simply applying a small amount of colour to the end of a cotton bud and rubbing it onto the client's skin, either behind the ear or on the inside of the elbow. Place a small plaster over where it has been rubbed and advise the client to notify you should there be any reaction. If there is nothing after 48 hours, the client will be fine to have colour applied.

Skin tests are a legal requirement of most salons these days, so as to cover any possible legal proceedings in the future. It is advised that all clients have this test done regardless, so that should they decide to have colour in the future, they don't have to wait for 48 hours. The test needs to be redone once a year to be on the safe side, and must be recorded and signed by the salon and the client.

a hairdresser is by the way you touch their hair, so do not be frightened to get your hands into the hair straightaway.

Remember during consultation that it is important to establish what you are doing to the hair, how long it will take and the cost. This will comfort the client and reassure them, as there is nothing worse than a client having their hair done and wondering the whole time how much it's all going to cost or how long they are expected to be there.

Always be polite to clients and explain exactly what you are doing to them. This makes the client feel more at ease and makes them feel as though you care. Most clients are also very interested to know what you are doing – after all it is their hair you are working on!

# consultation categories

To make the consultation process easier for you to remember, it has been divided into four categories that we will look at in detail. Each section is then broken down further to help you and your client work together to get the best results.

## History

It may seem excessive, but you really need to know everything your client has had done to their hair in the past, especially when it comes to using chemicals. Find out the following:

- ★ What chemicals have been on the hair?
- ★ Who has done it?
- ★ What haircuts have they had before?
- ★ Did they like them?
- ★ Have they had any reactions to chemicals?
- ★ Have they had any scalp problems?
- ★ What is on the hair now?
- ★ What products do they use?
- ★ Have they used any natural lightening products? ( e.g. Sprays to lighten hair in the sun – these contain chemicals that react to most other chemicals.)
- ★ What colours have they used that they have liked?
- ★ Have they ever had a perm, and did they like it?
- ★ Have they ever had an adverse result to a skin test?

Remember that hair grows approximately 1 cm (0.5 in) a month, so if the hair is 15 cm (6 in) long, it is approximately one year old. Bear this in mind when finding out what chemicals have been on the hair, as a lot can be done to hair during a year.

Asking these and many other questions about the hair's history can help you to achieve the best results. The history of the hair will help determine what colour you can or cannot use, what haircut would most suit them, and whether the hair is still affected by perms or any other chemical treatments that they may have had in the past. Remember to record any findings in a card index so as to make it easier for you or any other hairdresser in your salon the next time that client comes in. It also means that the client won't be asked the same questions every time!

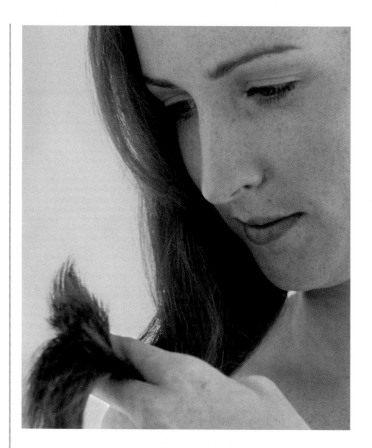

## Lifestyle

A client's lifestyle can play a big part in how their hair is. Everything from the cut to the colour you use can be affected by someone's job – after all, a lawyer and a fashion designer are unlikely to want to portray the same image. Lifestyle also plays a big part in the amount of time a client has to visit the salon and how often, not to mention how much time they have to style their hair at home.

It's a good idea to ask about a client's hobbies when it comes to both cutting and chemical work, as some people may play a lot of sports which can result in washing hair very regularly, possibly even more than once a day. If this is the case, having a haircut that needs to be restyled every time is

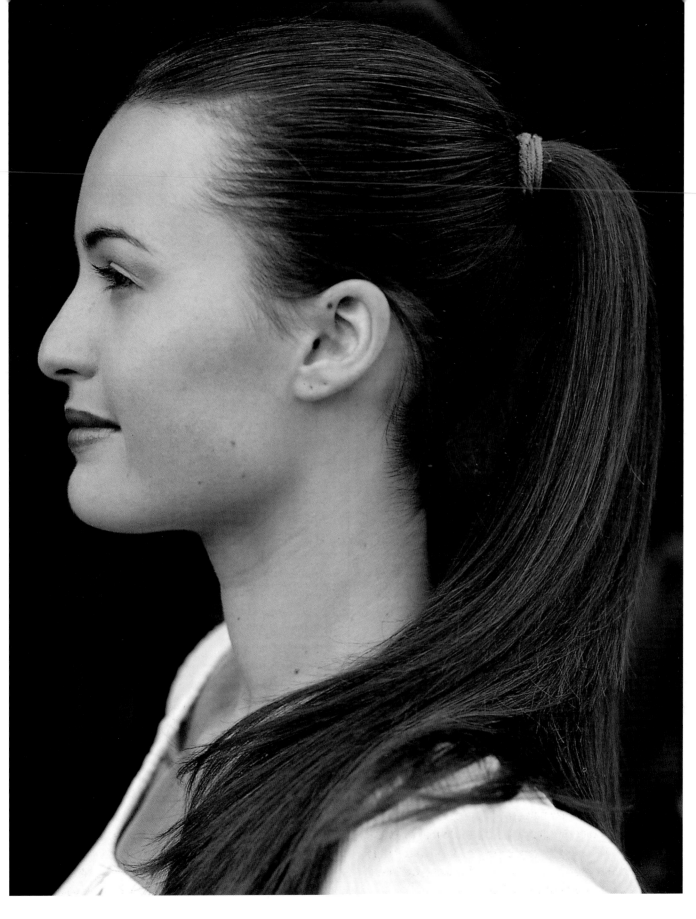

not such a great idea. Similarly, some colours fade more quickly than others or even disappear altogether if washed more regularly, so this will help you to decide on a more suitable cut and chemical products.

Budget fits into lifestyle in different ways. How much can the person afford when having their hair done? How often can they afford to come back and have it redone? And what budget do they have for the upkeep – can they afford to buy the products that will recreate the style created in the salon? When discussing budget with a client it is important that you take a subtle approach, as some clients may find it offensive or think that you are doubting their ability to pay. Question carefully and use tactful techniques.

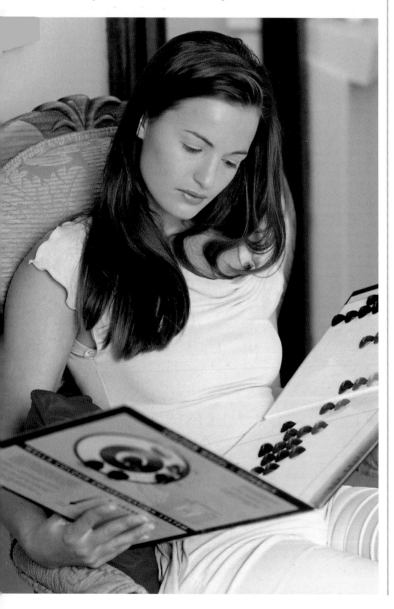

Important lifestyle questions to ask include:

★ Do they play sports?
★ How often do they wash their hair?
★ What do they do for a living?
★ How should their hair look for work?
★ How often can they come back to the salon?
★ How long have they got to spend in the salon at any one time?
★ How much time they can spend doing their own hair?
★ What is their budget?

## Using visuals

During consultation it is a good idea to use as many visual aids as possible; this will connect your vision with that of the client and make it easier to agree on an outcome based on the client's needs and wants.

Visuals can be from the client's past hair history – a client may bring photos of previous hairstyles that they have had and liked. These are probably the best sort of visual, as you know and the client knows that it is possible to create this look, as they have had it before.

Clients often like the look of famous people's hair or pictures of models in magazines. This is also a good visual in terms of knowing exactly what the client wants, but be aware that things such as hair type, texture or density can be completely different and make the look impossible to recreate. The client may have hair growth patterns which are not suitable for this look, or their face shape may not suit it. Be sensitive and tactful and approach it professionally: explain why the look won't work and give alternatives that are similar but that would suit them much more. This way the client knows that you are being honest and it is not that you cannot do the style.

If all else fails and they will not be dissuaded, always remember that the client is always right. You might disagree personally and professionally, but if they are set on a certain style you must do it. Be sure to warn them, however, that it may not turn out as they had hoped – at least then you are somewhat covered if they try to complain afterwards. It is a similar story with colour. Some colours do not suit certain skin tones while others do, but if a client wants it and the hair is in good enough condition and able to accept the colour without any problems, then you must follow their wishes. Again, it is their choice, and they are the ones who

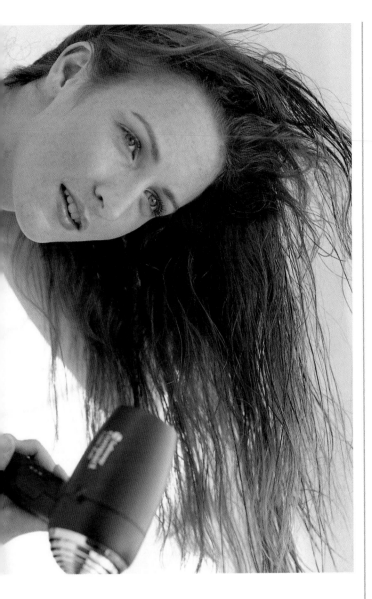

colour they have picked, it may not turn out as they had hoped. It is possible to be 100 per cent confident that you can achieve a precise colour, but it either takes a lot of experience and training or it involves becoming a professional specialist in colouring.

Visuals will always be one of the best ways of connecting with a client's image of what they want – just be aware of the challenges that go with them.

## Maintenance

Maintaining the look that you create for a client can be costly, and it is important to find out if your client can afford the time and money to do this. It's one thing creating a wonderful look for a client, but if it needs redoing every six weeks then they will soon go elsewhere for something more manageable. Ensure that your client's maintenance regime will fit the style, colour, perm, etc. that you are doing for them.

Maintaining a style at home is hard for most people, so to make sure that a client has a style that they can keep up, it's always best to find out in consultation what equipment they have at home and what they can handle doing themselves. Ask them the following questions:

★ Can they blow-dry?
★ Do they know how to use a brush to blow-dry?
★ What brushes do they have?
★ Do they leave the hair to dry naturally?

It is pointless having a style that needs blow-drying with a brush and hairdryer if the client does not own one, cannot use one or does not know how to use it properly. So when you come to decide a style, make sure that it fits the maintenance abilities of the client.

Some styling and chemical services require more extensive maintenance, such as special shampoos and conditioners or even treatments. Establish discreetly that the client can afford to purchase these, as they can be expensive. Similarly, some styles will require purchasing certain styling aids, possibly rollers, tongs or straightening irons. Make sure that they are willing to do this before giving them a style that they can't recreate without them. Regarding styling products in general, find out what they use and how often they use it; you may be able to advise them on what would best for them and their hair.

have to wear it. If you can lead them in another direction, though, you should – a bad colour decision from the client is not a great advert for you as a stylist!

Using colour charts is highly advised so that you are both agreed on the same colour. It is surprising how differently two people can view the same colour – your idea of red, for example, can be completely different to your client's idea of red. Using a colour chart will show you exactly what the client has in mind, but do bear in mind that the hair doesn't always come out the colour they have shown you. Many different factors determine how a colour will come out on someone's hair, so always warn clients prior to colouring that because of the hair condition or because of a previous colour, that although you will get as close as possible to the

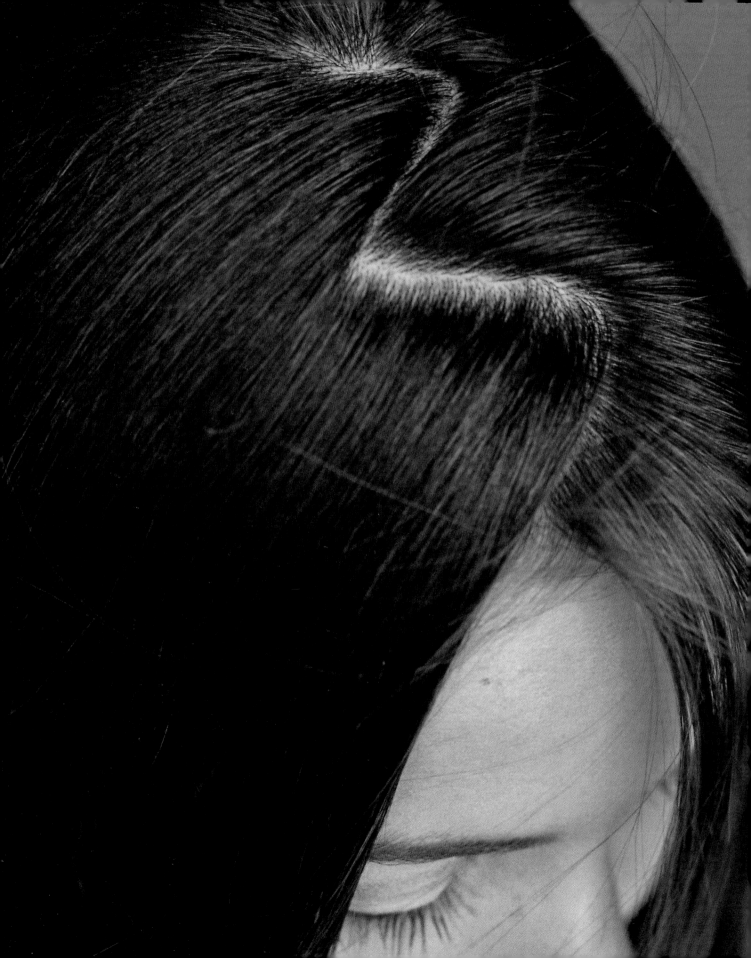

# 03 | down to the roots

# hair types and textures

Diagnosis of hair takes a lot of experience and practice and is split into different angles: type, texture, density and condition. It may seem straightforward, but if done incorrectly it can cause problems when it comes to chemicals. So let's break it up into sections and look at each one individually.

## Hair types

As a general rule our heritage and background, even from many generations back, determines the type of hair we have, as it is passed on via our genes. Hair types differ widely, from the Caucasian hair of most Europeans, to the afro hair of black people the world over. Asian hair is different again, but can share similar traits with apparently quite different hair. Chinese and Filipino hair, for instance, is very different but is usually very dark to black in colour and often strong hair. Similarly, Spanish, Italian and Swedish people have what looks like very different hair in colour, but the structure and density of the hair is similar. Identifying hair types is generally straightforward, and sometimes just looking at a person's face will give you clues.

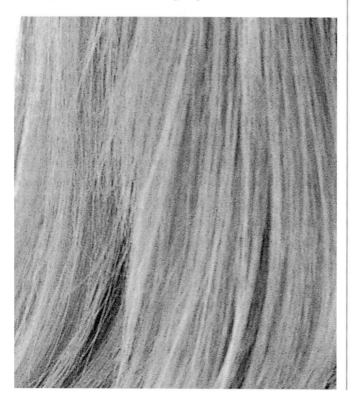

## Hair texture

Texture is usually identified in three categories: fine, medium or coarse. Be careful not to confuse the hair texture with the density or how much hair we have, which would be identified as thin, medium or thick. Texture is determined by the thickness of the individual strand of hair, whereas density is identified by how many hairs there are.

The diameter of an individual hair is generally bigger for coarse hair and smaller for fine. Coarse hair usually feels quite dry and can often, in Caucasian hair, be grey or white. Fine-textured hair is often soft and feels like a baby's hair. Be warned that fine hair is often easier to damage with chemicals or heat, as it does not have the same internal strength as medium or coarse hair. Medium hair is somewhere in the middle of fine and coarse. Get as much practice as you can in identifying the look and feel of different people's hair, so that you can start to determine which is which.

## Hair density

To determine the density of hair, you need to assess how much hair there is. If it is thick there is lots of it, and if thin it is easier to see the scalp. Medium is again somewhere in the middle of the two.

To assess density, part the hair anywhere in the middle area around the crown and see how dense the hair is coming out of the scalp. Be aware that you can have coarse hair that is thin in density, or have fine hair texture that is thick in density – i.e. you have a lot of it.

## Hair condition

Different lengths need to be looked at in order to be able to work out what the hair's condition is. For example, many people can have dry ends (from chemical or heat damage) and oily roots, so depending on the hair length look at the

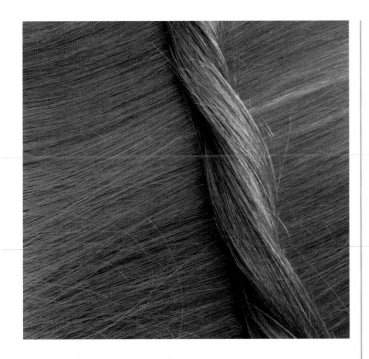

roots as one diagnosis and the ends as another. If the client has very long hair, you can also consider the middle sections as they could also be different. Below is a list of different hair conditions and a guide to the giveaway signs for easy diagnosis.

## OILY

Normally always at the root of the hair and very rarely at the ends. Oil through the lengths of the hair is eliminated by use of colour and heated appliances, which are both very common these days. Oily lengths can often look a little glossy, as oil makes hair look slick. Oil also makes hair limp, and you can struggle to get it to do anything. It is often thinner hair that has problems with oil – thicker hair tends to be more dry and brittle as not enough oil is created to make it supple.

## NORMAL

This is what everyone wants. Shiny, glossy, bouncy hair, which feels silky, and shines constantly. Not oily, no dryness – just perfect.

## DRY

There are two kinds of dryness, and many people confuse the two. One is dryness from lack of moisture, or oil, and the other type is hair that often feels dry from the damage that has been caused inside the hair's structure, normally called dry/damaged or sensitized hair. This sort of hair is also dry to the touch, but is often fragile, too, and breaks quite easily. There are tests which can identify this better (see elasticity testing on page 29).

If the hair structure is damaged, the hair is weakened. This makes the hair look dry, but if you use a reconstructing treatment (which is for strengthening hair) the dryness will also disappear, even though reconstructants are often in liquid form where conditioners for dryness come in cream form.

To recap, dry hair is caused by lack of moisture and external damage, and dry sensitized hair is caused by internal damage.

## COMBINATION

Combination hair is a mixture of the above, e.g. oily roots and dry ends; dry hair with dry sensitized ends; normal roots with dry ends, etc.

It is not possible to have oily ends and dry roots, as the oil secretes from the scalp first. Hair at the root is 'newer' fresh hair, whereas at the ends it can be years old and have had much done to it, thus drying it out.

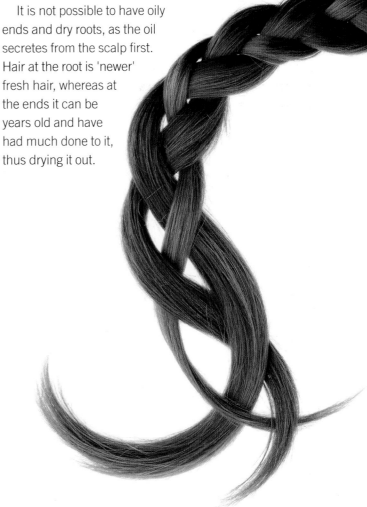

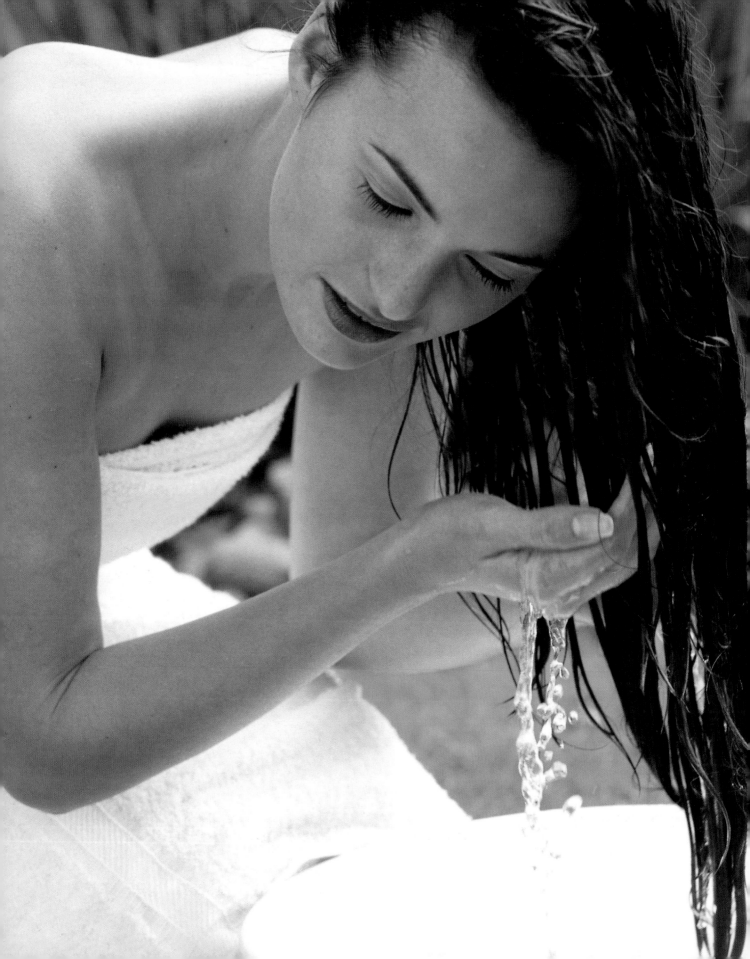

# How to care for different hair conditions

## OILY HAIR

Oil is secreted from the sebaceous glands in the scalp. It is actually vital, as without it our hair would be dry and brittle – think of it as a lubricant that puts some moisture on the hair. However, some people suffer from excess oil, and this can be a result of many things such as bad diet, hormones, puberty and sometimes medication. The result is that the sebaceous gland goes into overdrive and produces more than is needed, but there are ways to help slow it down.

Hot water tends to stimulate sebaceous glands, so when shampooing always use tepid or even cold water. Massage also over-stimulates the glands, and no matter how much you really want to scrub the scalp to get it clean, it's the worst thing you can do. Wet the hair and apply shampoo for oily hair, but use the flats of your hands, not the fingertips, to lightly rub the shampoo in, to avoid stimulating the glands unneccessarily. Another trick is to leave the shampoo on the hair for 3–5 minutes. This allows it to penetrate and clean the hair itself.

When using conditioner, if you have dry ends make sure to use the smallest amount and do not get it anywhere near the scalp, as it will just make the hair oily even more quickly than usual. There are other alternatives such as leave-in conditioners, which are a lot easier to apply to just the ends of the hair, and are often lighter in formula.

## DRY/SENSITIZED HAIR

Dry hair can tangle easily, especially when it is dry/sensitized, so when shampooing try not to make it even easier for the hair to tangle. You can rub the scalp firmly, but put your fingers into the hair and rotate the finger ends as opposed to moving the whole hand and fingers. A really invigorating scrubbing motion is to be avoided, as this will knot the hair.

On long hair always 'smooth shampoo', as long hair tangles easily and is hard to comb out afterwards. Smooth shampooing is like stroking the hair from root to tip in a massaging motion. You can work the shampoo in, but always work in the direction of growth to reduce knotting. Again, leaving the shampoo on the hair allows it to penetrate and cleanse, removing dirt from the hair itself.

## PROBLEM SCALPS

Dandruff comes in two types: oily and dry. Oily dandruff is just the same as dry, but if the sebaceous gland is producing too much oil the dandruff sticks to the scalp, as opposed to dry where it falls onto your shoulders. Oily dandruff is similar to cradle cap, which often occurs on baby's heads. With either type, using the fingertips to release the dandruff is a good idea, but be sure to keep your nails short. Work in small, circular movements and rotate the fingers, helping to release the dead skin. Using specially formulated shampoos can also help.

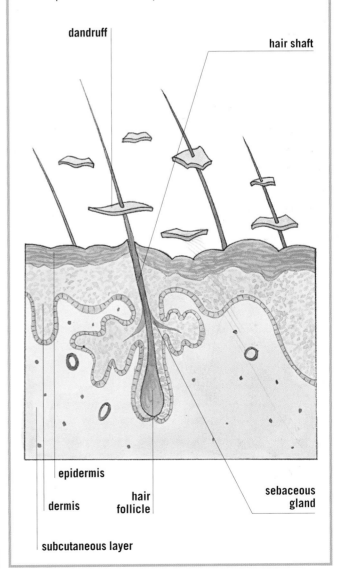

dandruff
hair shaft
epidermis
dermis
hair follicle
sebaceous gland
subcutaneous layer

# shampooing

An old wives' tale is that you should change your shampoo now and again, as your hair will get too used to it and it will no longer be effective. This is incorrect. It is not that your hair gets used to it; more that the shampoo has done the job that it was supposed to do. For instance, if you have dry hair and use the appropriate shampoo, in time it will moisturize the hair and eventually will probably be providing too much moisture for the hair, which is now 'normal'. And yes, it is possible to over-moisturize hair – it makes the hair either fly-away and static or very limp and lifeless.

## how to...

**SHAMPOO HAIR**

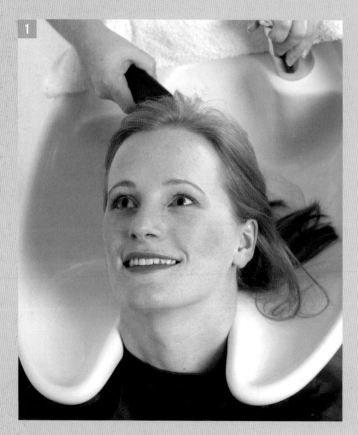

① Place a gown and towel on the client's shoulders. Place the client comfortably at the back wash, ensuring all their hair is in the basin.

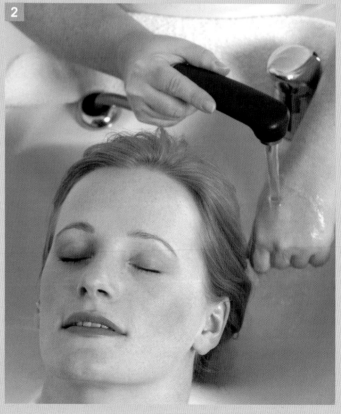

② Run the water on the back of your hand until it is at the desired temperature. Check that the water temperature is fine for the client by flashing it on to the back of their hair.

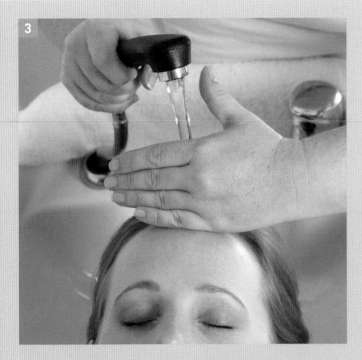

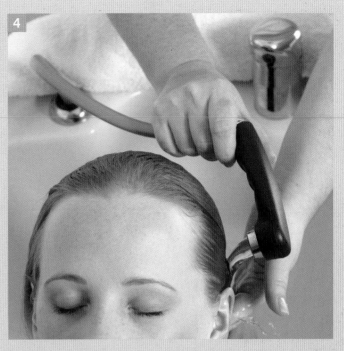

③ Hold the shower head in one hand and cup the other hand, placing it on the hairline to protect the face from water running down it. Start to run the shower head around the front hairline. The shower head should be held close to the head and just below the thumb of the hand protecting the client's face – use this hand as a protection barrier or to rub the hair to help the water penetrate.

④ When running the water around the face area, you can pull the protecting hand back with the shower head to help guide excess water around the face and hairline area. Once the top of the hair is wet, move the shower head around the back of the head.

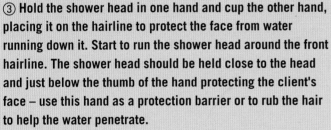

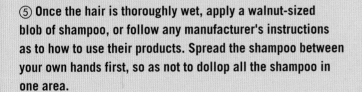

⑤ Once the hair is thoroughly wet, apply a walnut-sized blob of shampoo, or follow any manufacturer's instructions as to how to use their products. Spread the shampoo between your own hands first, so as not to dollop all the shampoo in one area.

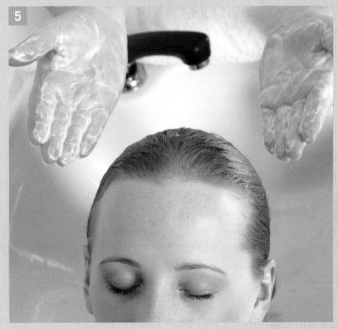

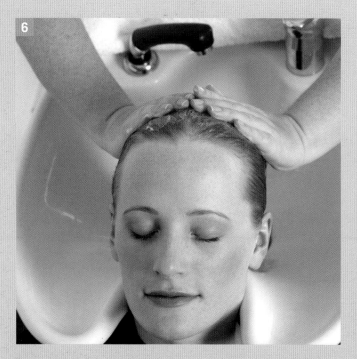

⑥ Lightly spread the shampoo from front to back and over the sides of the hair. Don't forget the underneath, near the neck. With a kneading motion, start at the hairline and work down towards the crown, then from ears to crown and from the crown down to the nape.

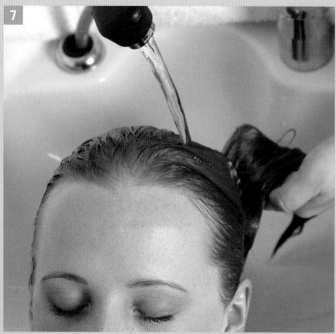

⑦ Once the shampoo is evenly distributed (it may not lather on first shampoo as it is picking up dirt first), rinse in the same manner as when wetting hair down.

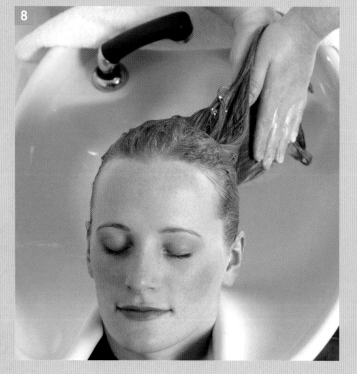

⑧ Re-shampoo as before. This time the shampoo should lather. Rinse as before, but this time rinse for longer and make sure to rub the hair a little while doing so to remove all shampoo. A good trick to remove all shampoo is to rub the hair without water as if you were shampooing it. This will bring the last lather up, at which point you can rinse again.

Now you are ready for conditioning.

# conditioning and treating

Conditioners come in many different forms, from mousses and lotions to creams and sprays, both rinse-out and leave-in. Leave-in conditioner is normally lighter in formula, yet most people seem to think that it leaves the hair heavier. This is untrue – it is very good for fine or thin hair, particularly as it is normally a spray rather than a cream.

Leave-in conditioners do come in creams as well, and these can be used to help extra-dry hair after using a rinse-out conditioner, and can also help to smooth curly hair that is going to be dried straight.

It is not always a good idea to massage conditioner into the scalp (unless, of course, it is made specifically to go on the scalp) as it can make the hair very limp and can cause the hair to become oily more quickly. When applying rinse-out conditioners, always use just the recommended amount and spread it evenly through the lengths of the hair only. If

the hair is short, then put the conditioner on the back of your hand, dab your fingers to get a trace of it on your fingertips, then carefully rub it into the ends. You will find that short hair often doesn't need conditioner as badly as longer hair, as it tends to be less damaged and fresher.

If you are using the correct shampoo, the shampoo should treat the hair as well. Always remember that it is not just conditioner that helps to moisturize dry hair – using the appropriate shampoo (oily, dry, dandruff eliminating, damaged, coloured, etc.) will also help to care for hair.

## how to...

### CONDITION HAIR

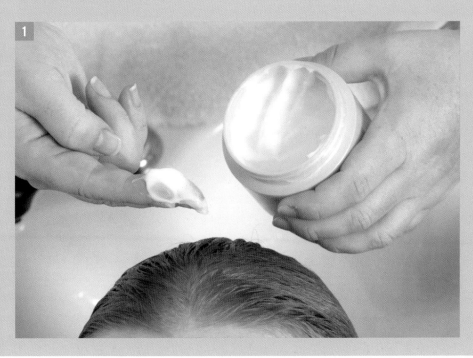

① After two shampoos, remove any excess water with a towel. Be careful to blot only – do not rub dry as this is more likely to damage and knot the hair. Measure out about a walnut-sized blob of conditioner into your palm or the back of your hand.

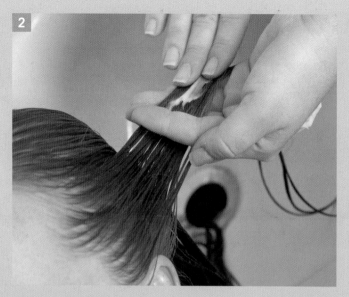

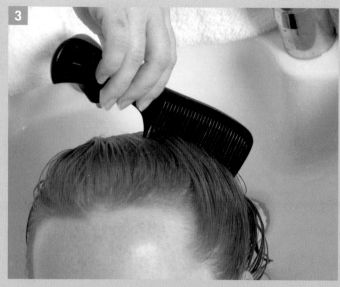

② Starting with one side, take small handfuls of hair and apply a small amount of the conditioner to it. Work into the hair in a downwards movement to the ends. Remember only to apply to the ends, or the mid-lengths and ends, depending on the length. Work through the hair, section by section, doing the same thing until you have covered all the ends.

③ Using a wide-tooth comb, gently comb out the knots starting at the ends and working up. Note that if you have used more than the recommended amount of conditioner, when you comb the hair there will be excess conditioner which will spread to the roots. A walnut-sized amount is enough to condition most long hair, so use less if the hair is shorter.

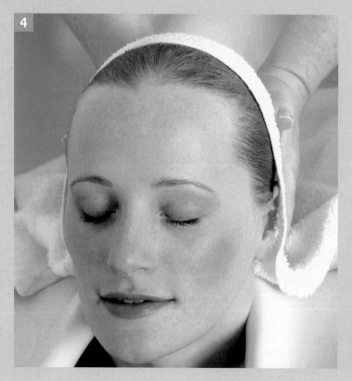

## tip

Hair is a lot more vulnerable and easier to damage when wet, so be gentle when combing hair. Always comb from the ends up to the roots in small segments, never from the roots down, as all the knots will gather in one area and are then very hard to remove. This is only necessary for hair of 8 cm (3 in) or more, as shorter hair does not get as tangled when combing.

④ Once combed through, rinse the hair thoroughly and then towel dry. Conditioner is hard to remove completely if too much is used, so again – use the correct amount, which is probably less than you think.

## Treatments

Treatments come in many different forms – from moisturizing and colour-saving, to after-sun and conditioning. Most help to improve the internal strength and build of the hair and come in the form of heavy creams, although professional treatments sometimes come in a spray formula. These do not look like they have much power, but they do, and because they are a spray they infuse well into the hair. When using a cream, again you do not need masses of product, so always follow the recommended amount even if it doesn't look as if it is enough. Sprays usually come in individual applications, so use it all.

## how to...

### APPLY TREATMENT TO HAIR

When using treatments, you do not need to apply a conditioner before or after; a treatment is like an intensive conditioner, and they are often a reconstructant which actually rebuilds the hair's strength from the inside whilst also making quite a difference to the outer appearance. They will generally make hair easier to manage, soft and shiny.

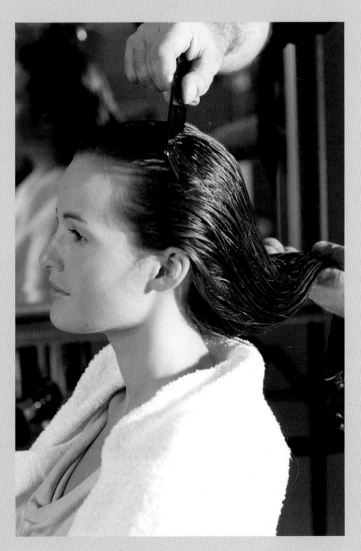

① **Shampoo hair twice with an appropriate shampoo.**

② **Using a towel, blot the hair as much as you can. The more water you can get out of the hair, the less diluted the treatment is.**

③ **Sit the client away from the back wash at a section. Clip the hair into four sections by parting the hair down the middle from front to nape, then from ear to ear, creating a hot-cross bun effect across the head. Clip each section up loosely.**

④ **Take sub-sections and apply the treatment to mid-lengths and ends of hair (depending on length). Work in a downwards motion away from the scalp, working the treatment in.**

⑤ **Take a wide-tooth comb and comb through each sub-section, from the ends up to the roots. Most treatments require leaving on for 10 minutes or so – in a salon a heat machine should be applied to enable the treatment to penetrate, but at home clingfilm wrapped around your hair and a hot towel will work just as well.**

# massage techniques

Massage can be the most relaxing part of having your hair done. It is often missed out, as salons are too busy, but it can make all the difference to a client's experience. A head massage can start even before a hair wash and does not need to be done just on wet hair. Proper scalp massages should only be done with a conditioner or a scalp treatment such as those for dandruff, psoriasis or environmentally-formed itchy scalp, caused by dirt and pollution.

## how to...

### PERFORM A HEAD MASSAGE – STAGE ONE

To start a relaxation massage for a client who has just entered the salon, sit the client in a quiet area or another room altogether, if you have a relaxation room. Explain to the client what you are doing as they may not be familiar with this service.

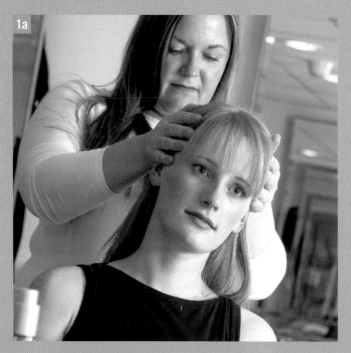
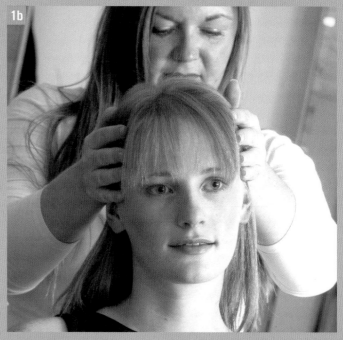

①ab **Place the palms of each hand on either side of the head and ask the client to relax. Slowly try to take control of the head's movement by rolling the head from side to side. Let the weight of the head be in your hands and the movement come from you, not the client. This is very relaxing and will** help the client to slow down. It may feel odd for some people at first, but with their eyes shut and peace around them – perhaps even some soft music playing and some candles or incense burning – they will soon be in a much happier frame of mind.

## STAGE TWO

The second stage of massage should be done at the back wash during the second shampoo, or if the conditioner/treatment is suitable for the scalp, you can massage during conditioning.

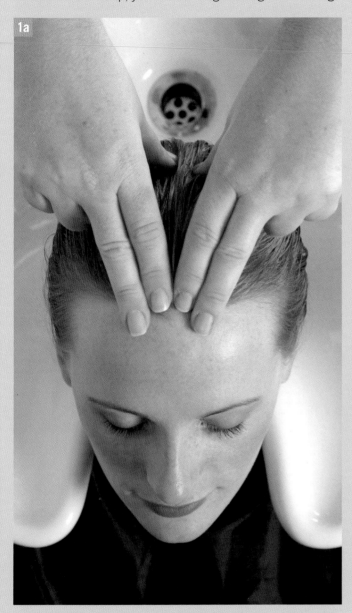

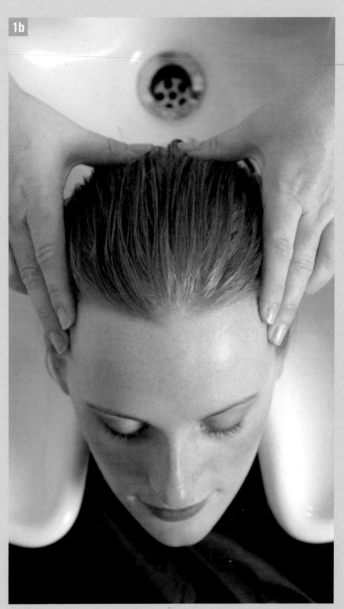

①ab **Start at the front of the head on the hairline, using slow, small circular movements with the fingertips and working back in a straight line towards the crown. Without losing contact from the client's head (as this breaks the** relaxing feeling), **move the fingers back one hand at a time to the start point and then work in the same motion towards the ears, working slowly around the hairline.**

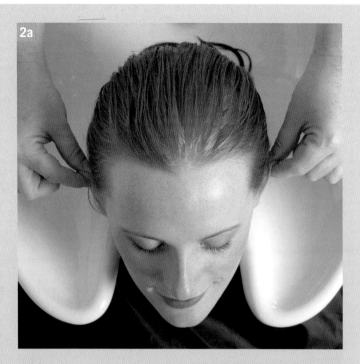

2a

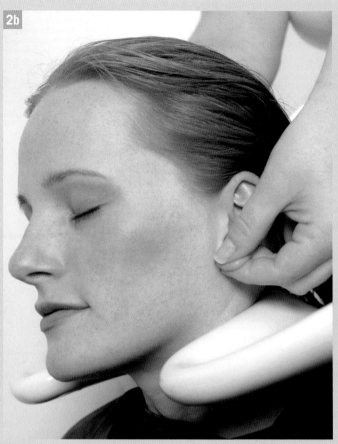

2b

②ab **The next stage again may feel odd for the client, but is very relaxing. Once at the ears, do not break contact, but with forefinger and thumb take hold of the top of the ear and slowly, in circular motions, move down the edge of the ear until you reach the lobe. Tug the lobes very lightly.**

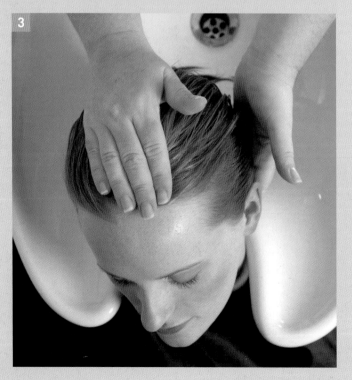

3

③ **Again without breaking contact, move in circular movements behind the ear and follow the hairline down to the nape. Once at the nape, take one hand off and hold the head steady at the top by placing your palm down gently on top of the head. Using the other hand, cup the neck into your hand and in a soft nipping motion, knead the neck. Next, slowly work all your fingertips up the back of the head in circular motions on both sides until at the crown. Working from the front hairline, do the same across both sides on the front. Gradually start to stroke the hair and finish with lightly pulling the fingers like a comb through the hair's lengths and ends.**

## STAGE THREE

The third part of the massage should be done once hair is washed and towel-dried. Put both hands together and with a light chopping motion, chop lightly onto the head starting at the top and working down the sides and back. This should only be done for about 10–20 seconds, as it is a relief massage to wake and stimulate after all the relaxing.

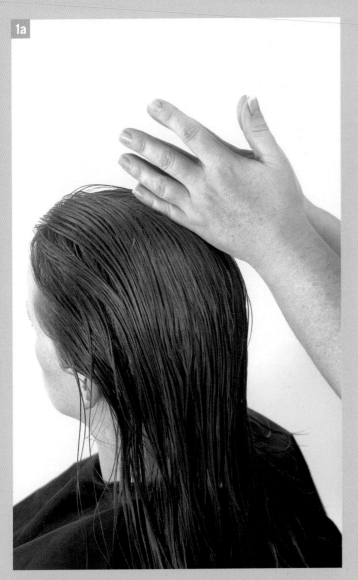

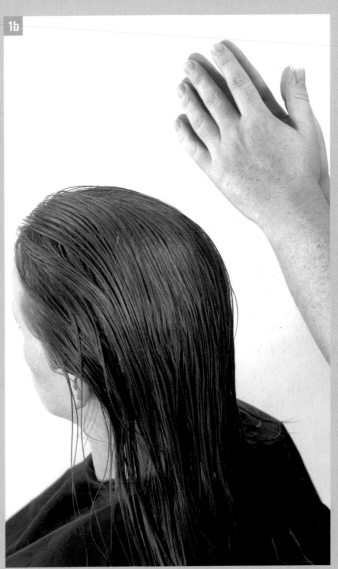

①ab **Chop lightly on the top, sides and back of the head. Like some other parts of the massage, this may well feel strange to the client at first. It is actually a very pleasant way** to be re-invigorated after the relaxation of the shampooing and conditioning, and your regular clients will not need to be persuaded to have it done.

# cutting hair: the basics

There are many factors to take into consideration when cutting different styles, but some things are universal whatever the cut. The following cutting techniques can be used on many styles, and sectioning is a vital skill to master.

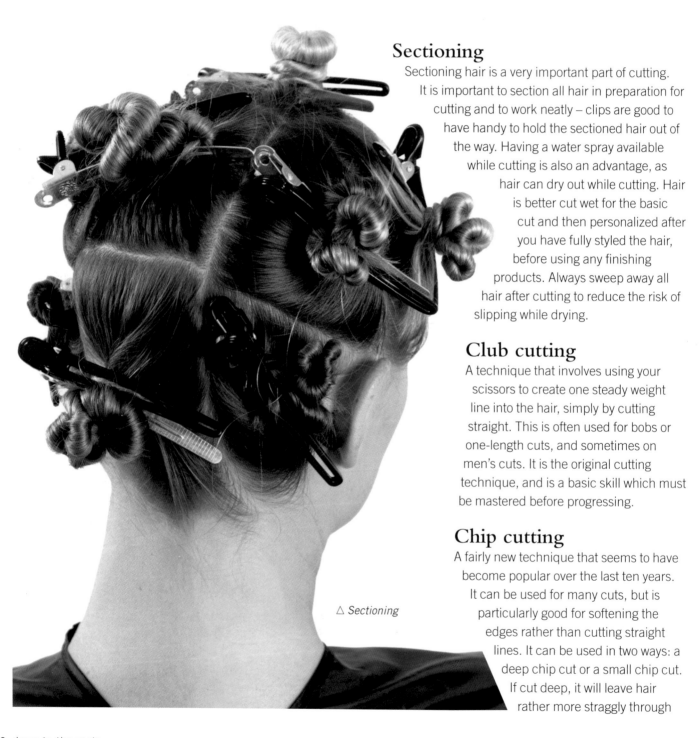

△ Sectioning

## Sectioning

Sectioning hair is a very important part of cutting. It is important to section all hair in preparation for cutting and to work neatly – clips are good to have handy to hold the sectioned hair out of the way. Having a water spray available while cutting is also an advantage, as hair can dry out while cutting. Hair is better cut wet for the basic cut and then personalized after you have fully styled the hair, before using any finishing products. Always sweep away all hair after cutting to reduce the risk of slipping while drying.

## Club cutting

A technique that involves using your scissors to create one steady weight line into the hair, simply by cutting straight. This is often used for bobs or one-length cuts, and sometimes on men's cuts. It is the original cutting technique, and is a basic skill which must be mastered before progressing.

## Chip cutting

A fairly new technique that seems to have become popular over the last ten years. It can be used for many cuts, but is particularly good for softening the edges rather than cutting straight lines. It can be used in two ways: a deep chip cut or a small chip cut. If cut deep, it will leave hair rather more straggly through

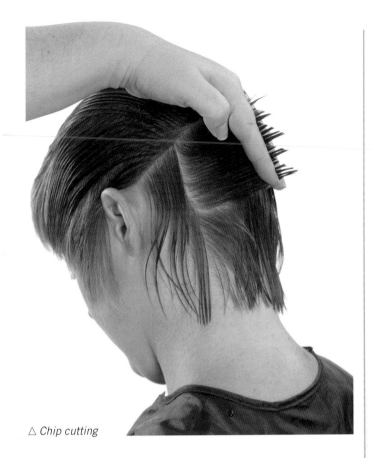

*△ Chip cutting*

## Channel cutting

A technique that involves the scissors cutting while sliding over hair that is laid flat; you don't pick up the hair in a section. This is always done on dry hair and normally on hair with layers in it, again to remove weight and put a sliced cut into the hairstyle. Never start channel cutting too far up the head, as it can cause hair to be cut too short and stand out.

## Slicing

Removes weight and bulk from the hair, but your scissors need to be very sharp for this. If not, they pull the hair and can cause damage to the hair's structure. This technique has a similar effect to the old-fashioned thinning scissors, as it makes some hairs shorter, therefore thinning the hair or creating some softness and slices. The difference is that with slicing, it is done as and where you see weight that needs removing, or where you wish to soften and add slices to the hair. It is also only in small amounts, whereas thinning scissors cut the whole section and do not quite give the same effect of softness.

*▽ Slicing*

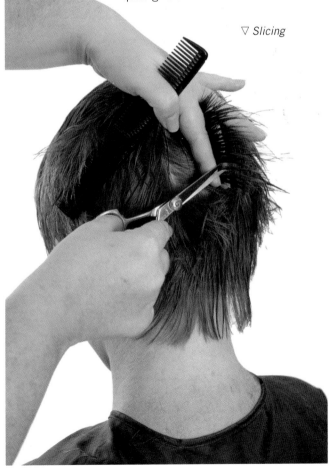

the ends, making it look like it does when it has grown out slightly. A smaller chip helps to soften a cut and creates some texture around the basic cut, instead of in straight lines or heavy edges.

## Scissor over comb

Used to remove weight in shorter hair, normally in the neck area and occasionally on sides when cut shorter into the ears, especially on men's hair. This technique takes a lot of practice to master. What happens is that the comb is moved very slowly following the shape of the cut (which normally follows the contours of the head shape) and the scissors cut over the top of the comb, taking out excess weight or hair that looks longer than the rest.

You can use this technique together with chipping on mid-length hair, still removing weight but using a soft chipping cut to create texture. It is not advised to do this chipping technique on hair that is fine or thin, as marks or lines in the haircut can appear unless you are aiming for a choppy, textured cut. Practice definitely makes perfect with this cut, and it can take many years to master it fully – practicing on a doll's head may help!

# the one-length cut

One-length cuts can be the hardest or the easiest of cuts, depending on the length of the hair and where it sits. Most one-lengths are cut in a similar way, however, and can be personalized afterwards using various other techniques.

## how to...

### CUT A ONE-LENGTH

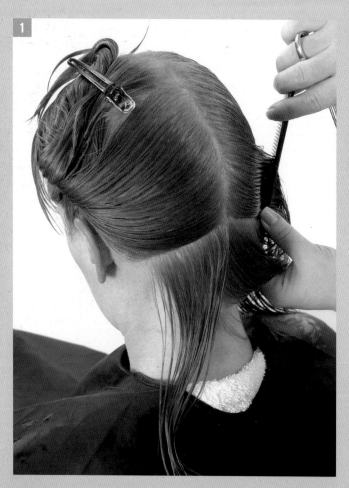

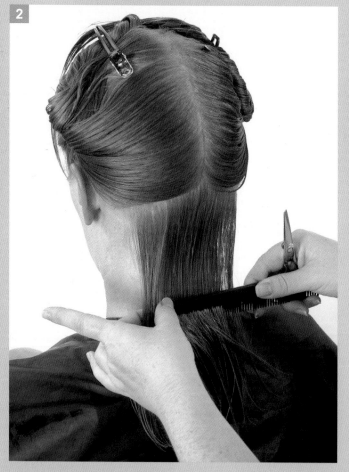

① Make sure any collars or capes are flat and well-fitted around the neck. Part the hair down the centre from front to nape. Take a sub-section going across the head from the centre part to the side and pin the rest of hair out of the way. Do the same to the other side.

② Comb the hair down tight into the neck – do not raise away from the neck, as you will get graduation in the hair cut and not have a solid one-length.

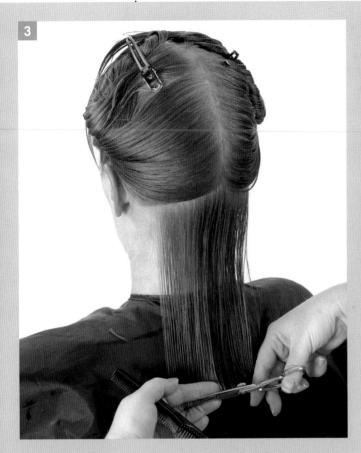

③ Cut straight across at the desired height and check both sides with your fingers to make sure the length is the same.

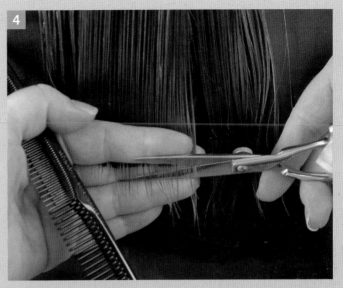

④ Take the next sub-section across the same way, from the centre part to the side, and pin the rest of the hair out of the way. Make sure the sub-sections are no wider than 1 cm (0.5 in), as you can lose length by cutting to the guide line from the last section. Continue this sub-section technique until reaching the crown.

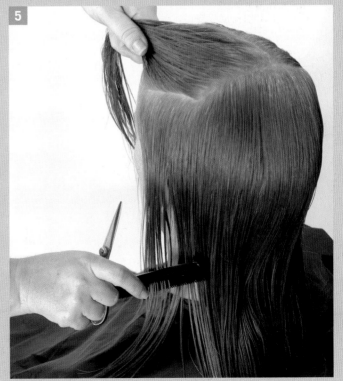

⑤ Take a sub-section from about 1–2 cm (0.5–1 in) above the ear, straight across.

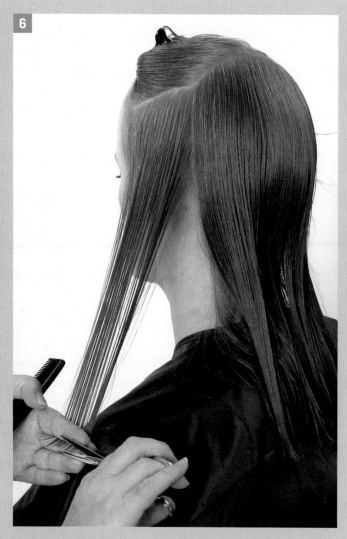

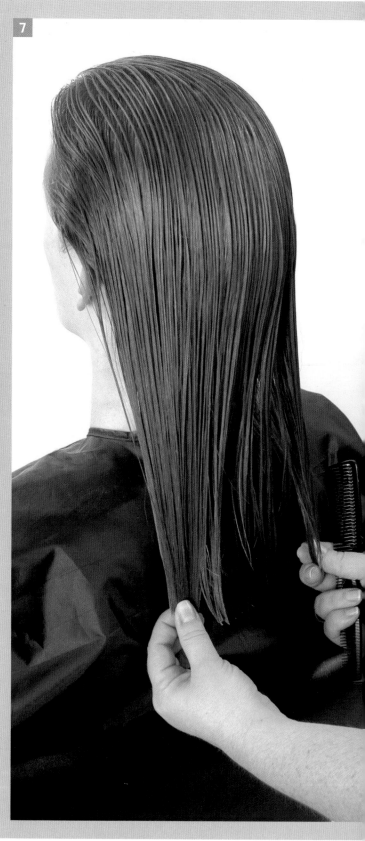

⑥ Take a piece of hair closest to the back of the ear of the sub-section, blend it into some of the hair already cut from the back sections, pull down in the same manner and cut to the same length. Try not to over-angle the fingers for cutting, or the hair will slope up at the front instead of being the same length.

Do the same on both sides of the head, but be sure to check that both sides are same length after each cut. Take the same sections right up to the centre parting.

⑦ Once finished, re-check the length by combing all the hair back behind the ears and down straight at the back. Soften the front by personalizing, if necessary.

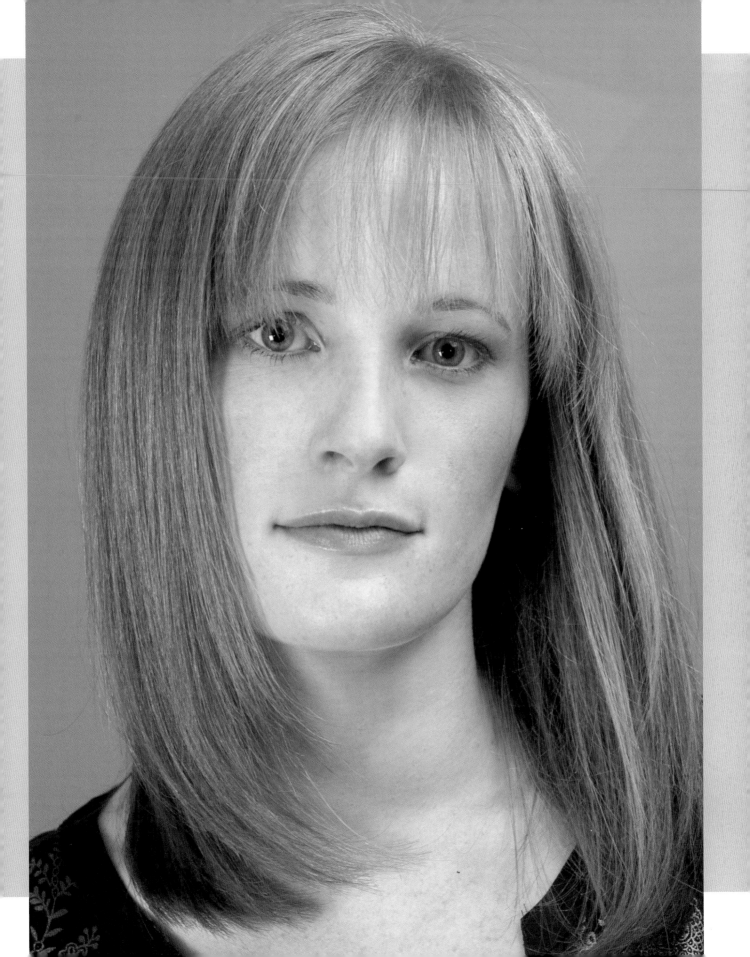

# the short cut

Short cuts have so much versatility and can be done in a variety of different ways. As with the one-length, there is much scope for personalizing the cut after it is done. Be sure to consult with your client before you do this, however, as they may like it styled a certain way.

## how to...

### CUT A SHORT STYLE

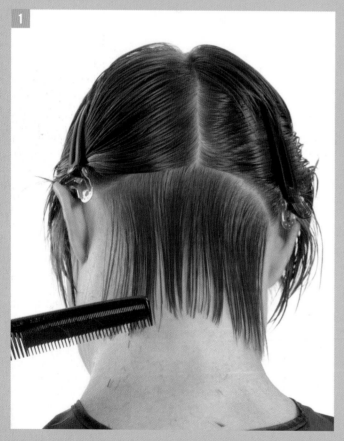

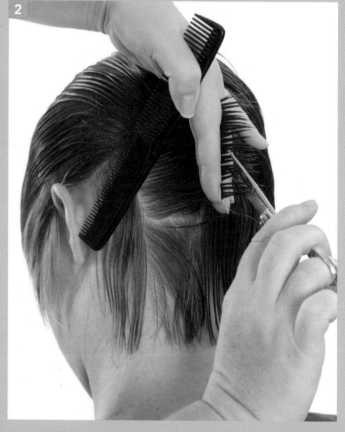

① Part the hair down the centre from front to nape. Subsection across about 2.5 cm (1 in) thick on either side and trim to the desired length.

② Take a vertical section down the middle area and pull the hair out to a 90 degree angle, straight out from the head. Using a chipping cut, cut the amount required out of the ends of the hair. Do the same through all of the sub-section, following the natural head shape round. Be careful not to pull all the hair out to the middle of the back section.

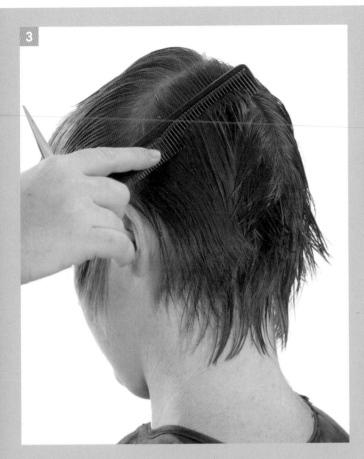

③ Once all the first section is complete, take a new horizontal section on both sides from the centre part, again about 2.5 cm (1 in) thick.

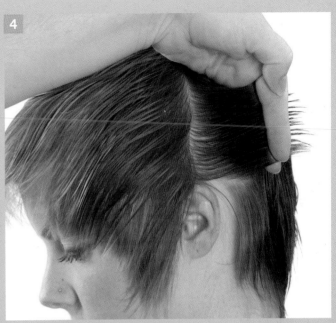

④ Divide into a vertical section, joining with the last cut for a guideline as to how much to remove. Pull out the section again at 90 degrees and chip the ends – remember, the deeper the chip, the more choppy the haircut. Repeat this process until reaching just below the crown area.

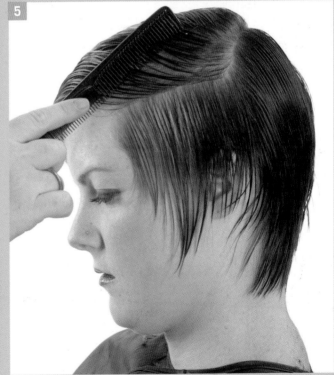

⑤ Moving on to the sides, take a section from just behind the ear about 2.5 cm (1 in) thick and part horizontally towards the front of the hairline, in front of the ear.

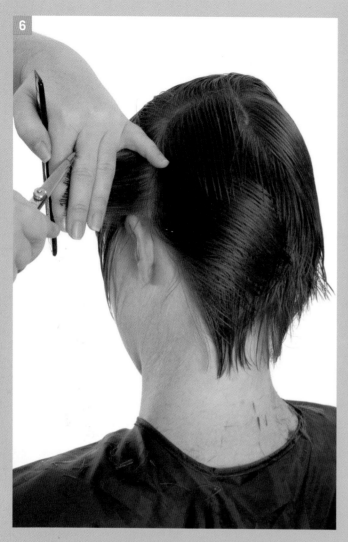

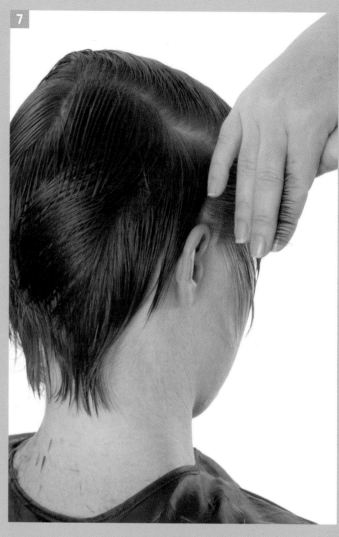

⑥ Take this section into smaller, vertical sub-sections, starting at the back of the ear and blending with some of the hair already cut from behind the ear to use as a guideline for length. Chip the ends to the length required.

⑦ Do the same on both sides of the head, but be sure to check that both sides are same length after each cut by pulling the hair out and visually checking. Take the same sections right up to the centre parting.

## tip

Never measure a cut by using a client's ears as a guideline – they are not always positioned at the same height on the head, and can even be different sizes altogether.

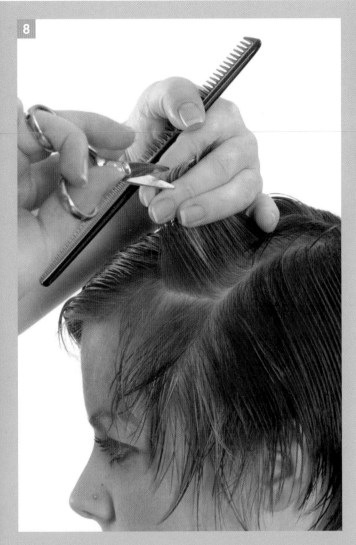

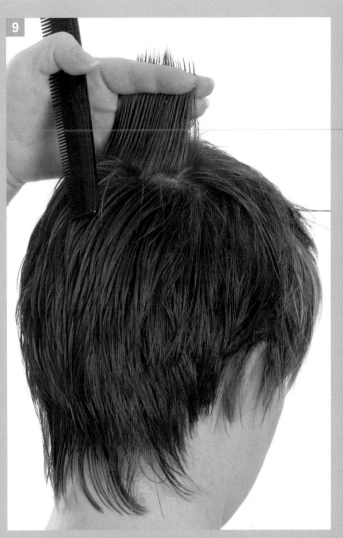

⑧ Going back to the first side, take another section horizontally from behind the ear going forwards, again no thicker than 2.5 cm (1 in). Pull out at a 90 degree angle from the head and chip out the required length. Repeat on the other side, and continue until you reach the hairline at the front.

⑨ Now take a section at the crown, rectangular in shape, from where you just finished cutting on the sides across the head to the other side. Again, this section should be no thicker than 2.5 cm (1 in).

▷

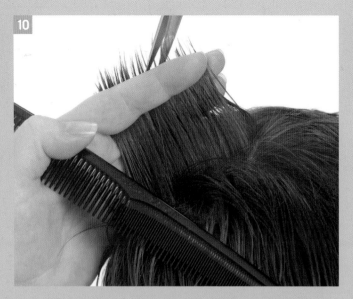

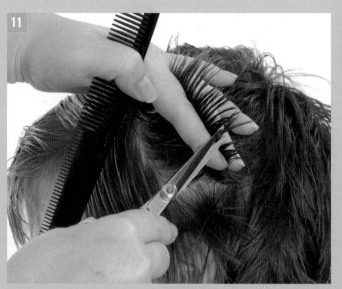

⑩ Cut a guideline by chipping to the length you require, bearing in mind the length you have cut the rest of the hair to. Follow this forward until about 2.5–5 cm (1–2 in) from the hairline at the front. Use each bit just cut as a guideline while cutting, and always pull straight up from the head. Work the last inch or so in the same fashion, but gradually leave a little more length so to create shape at the front.

⑪ Once all these sections are cut, there will be a horseshoe shape from the hairline with a triangular edge that will be un-cut. Take these sections and work round, chipping out the hair that is left long between your guidelines from the sides and back. In other words, there will be short hair on either side of the section you hold, and long hair in the middle to be cut out.

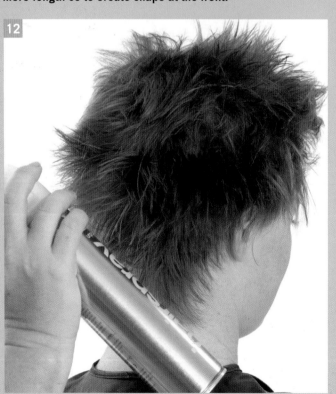

⑫ Once all the hair is cut, power dry and style. Personalize the cut using slicing and further chipping once styled to see where weight is still present.

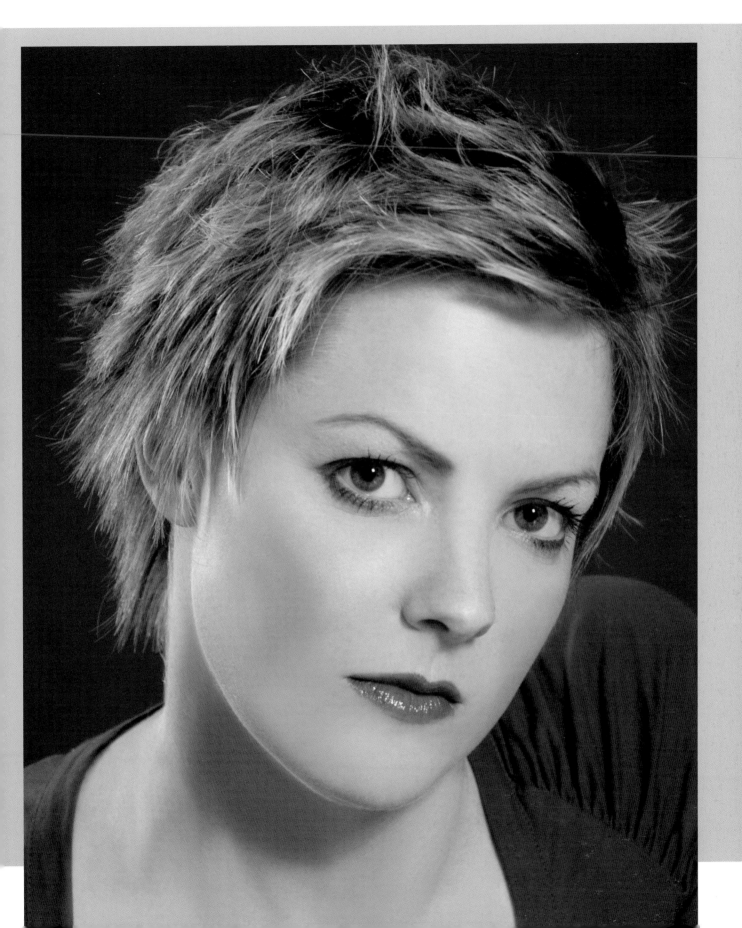

# the long graduation

A long graduation is essentially a one-length cut with soft graduation cut around the face to give shape and softness. Again, this cut can be personalized to make it individual, depending on the client's wishes.

## how to...

### CUT A LONG GRADUATION

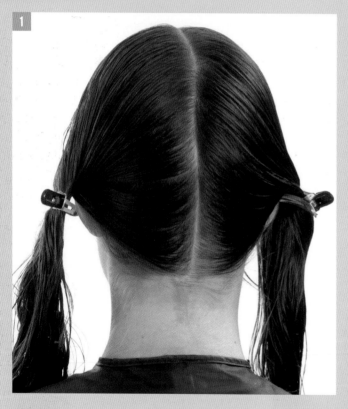

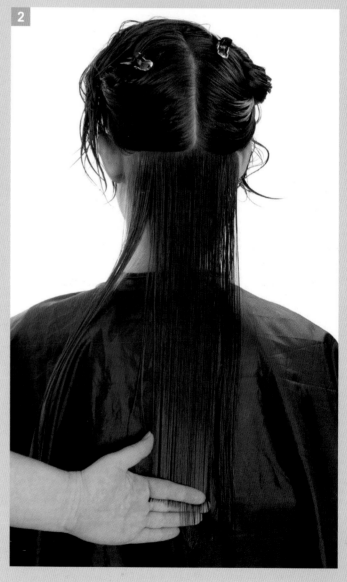

① Make sure any collars or capes are flat and well-fitted around the neck. Part the hair down the centre from front to nape.

② Take a sub-section going across from the centre parting to the side and pin the rest of the hair out of the way. Do the same to the other side. Comb the hair down tight into the neck. Cut straight across at the appropriate level and check both sides with your fingers to make sure the length is the same.

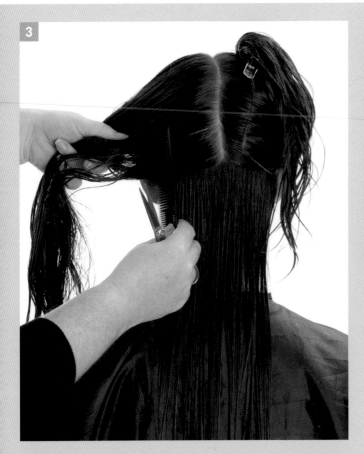

**3** Take the next sub-section across the same way, from centre part to side on either side, and pin the rest of the hair out of the way. Make sure that the sub-sections are no wider than 1 cm (0.5 in), as you can lose length by cutting to the guideline from the last section. Continue this sub-section technique until you reach the crown.

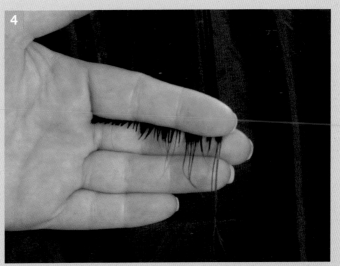

**4** Take a sub-section from about 1–2 cm (0.5–1 in) above the ear, straight across. Firstly take a piece of hair closest to the back of the ear and blend it into some of the hair already cut from the back sections. Pull it down and cut it to the same length. Try not to over-angle the fingers for cutting, or the hair will slope up at the front instead of being the same length. Follow this on both sides of the head but check both sides are same length after each cut.

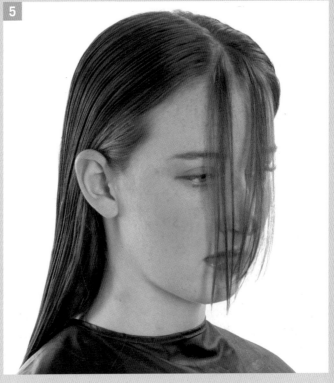

**5** Re-check the length by combing all the hair back behind the ears and down straight at the back. Now re-part the hair down the centre to the crown and comb the hair down to the back and sides as appropriate.

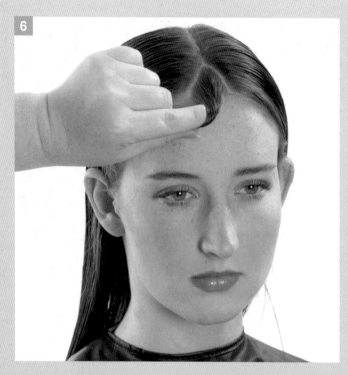

⑥ Draw an imaginary line from the middle of each eyebrow back into the hair, and take a small triangle at the very front of the hair in the centre. This hair will be your guideline for the shortest length of hair on the forward graduation.

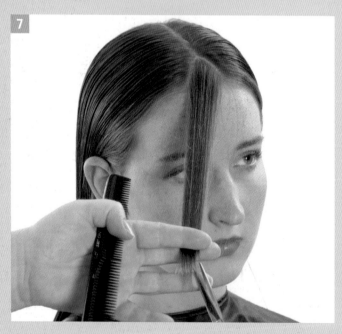

⑦ Chip this hair to the length required by your client. If the hair is curly, be aware that it will jump up shorter when dry.

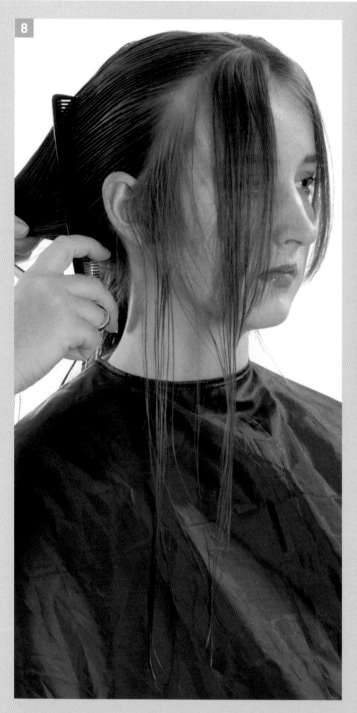

⑧ Once cut, take a section from the middle part down to the top of the ear, making the section no wider that 1–2 cm (0.5–1 in).

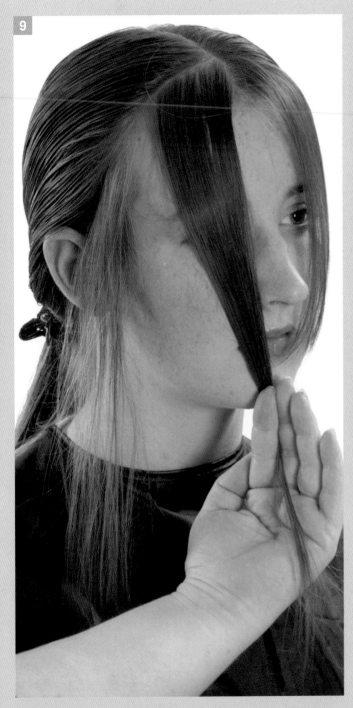

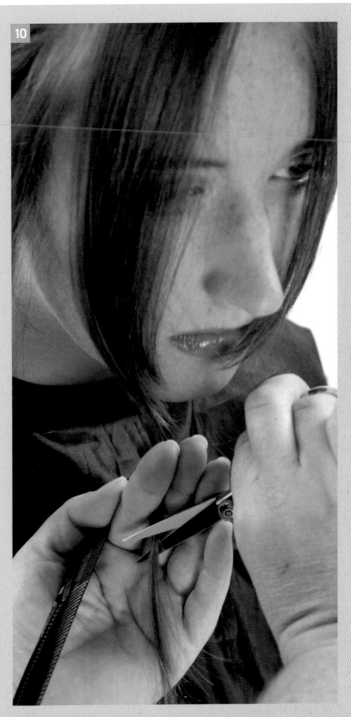

⑨ Imagine a line down the middle of the face and comb the section to that line. Cut on that line using the short guideline cut just done. Do this for the whole section, but the further down the section you get, the further down the imaginary line on the face you should cut.

⑩ Take the same section on the other side and cut in the same way, ensuring that you always cut to the imaginary centre line and that the shortest point is the guideline cut, getting longer as you move down the section.

▷

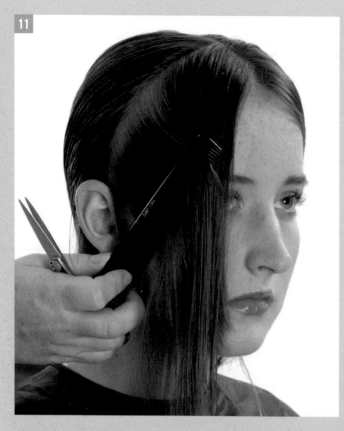

⑪ On the first side, take another section on the same angle, working back another 2 cm (1 in). Follow the guideline and imaginary centre line in the same way, cutting hair into the centre. Follow on the other side.

⑫ This technique can be worked right back into the centre part at the back of the head, or to create some soft layers in the back to blend, or it can be taken just to the top or back of the ear to create only forward graduation on the face

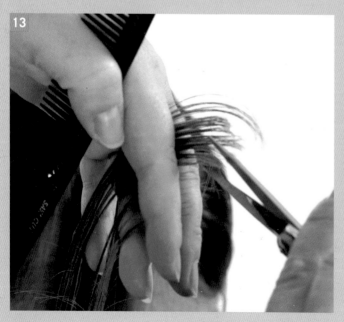

⑬ Once completed on both sides, blow-dry straight if possible, as it is easier to check the weight distribution. Once dried, remove any excess weight or uneven length in the graduation by slicing or chipping

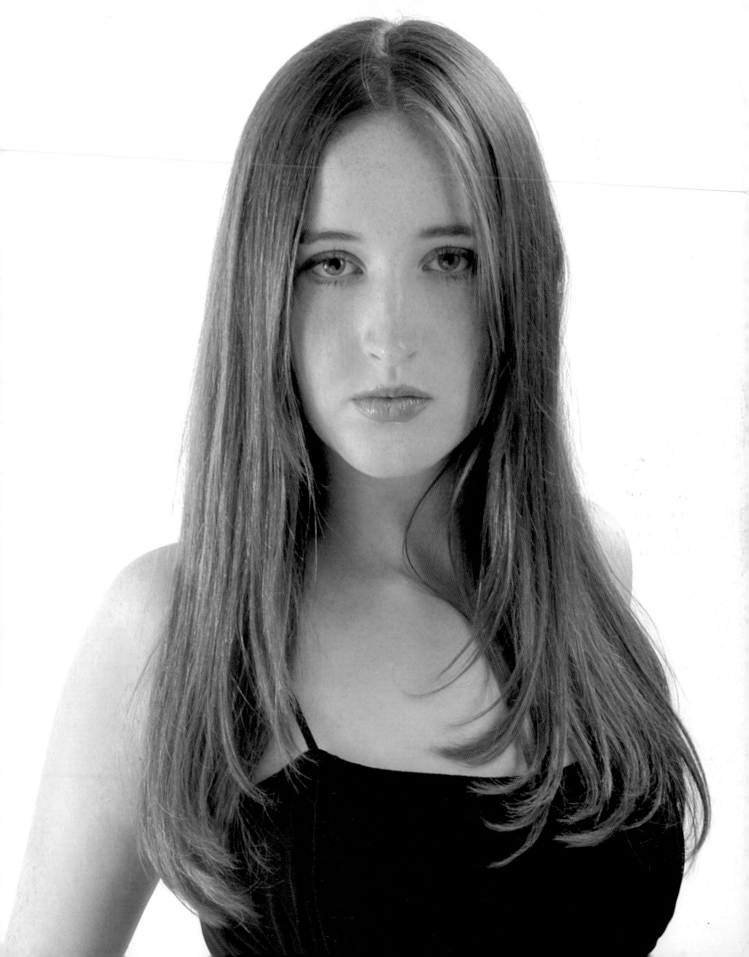

# the layered cut

Layers can come in many shapes and forms: round, universal, square and soft, to name but a few, with a different technique for each. This cut is a disconnected layer, which was done in order to keep the length but create shape.

## how to...

### CUT A LAYERED STYLE

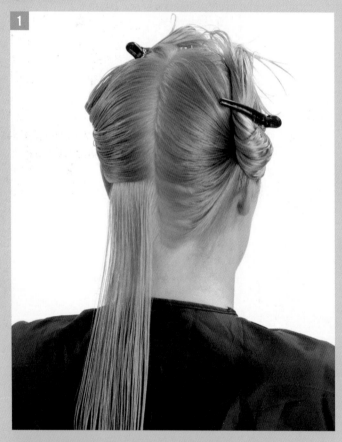

① Make sure any collars or capes are flat and well-fitted around the neck. Part the hair down the centre from front to nape, then take a sub-section going across from the centre part to the side and pin the rest of the hair out of the way.

② Do the same to the other side, combing the hair down tight into the neck. Cut straight across at the appropriate height.

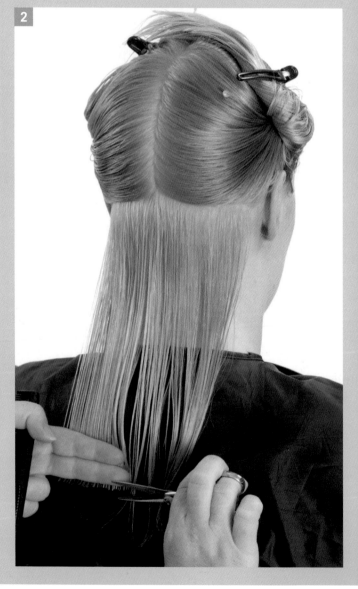

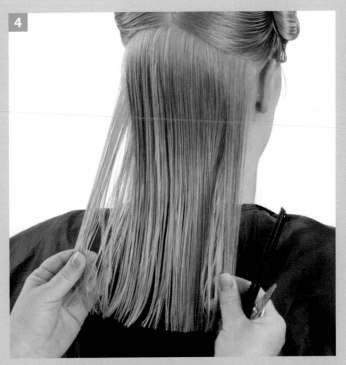

④ **Check both sides with your fingers to make sure that the length is the same, then continue this sub-section technique until reaching the crown.**

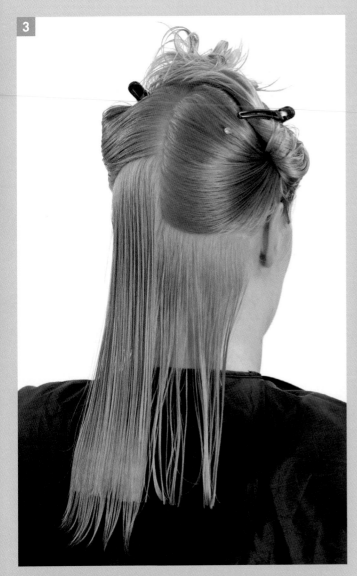

③ Take the next sub-section across the same way from the centre part to the side (on both sides) and pin the rest of the hair out of the way. Make sure that the sub-sections aren't too wide, as you can lose too much length this way.

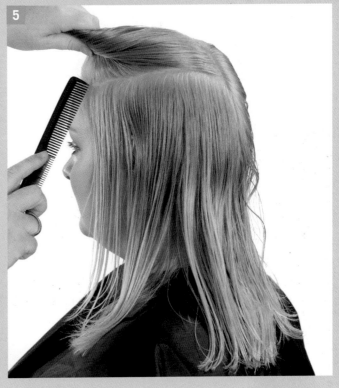

⑤ Take a sub-section from about 5 cm (2 in) above the ear, straight across. Blend some hair from the back of the section into some of the hair already cut from the back sections, then pull down as before and cut to the same length. Try not to over-angle the fingers for cutting, or the hair will slope up at the front instead of being the same length.

▷

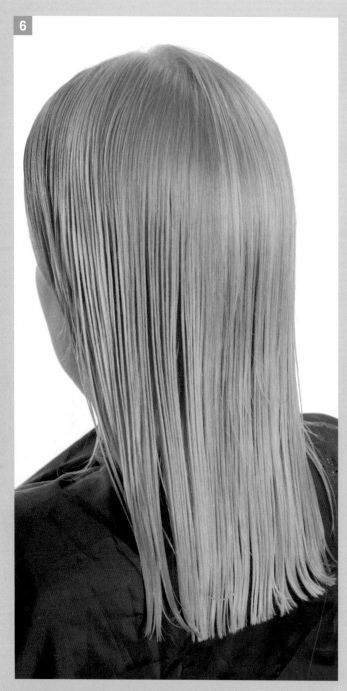

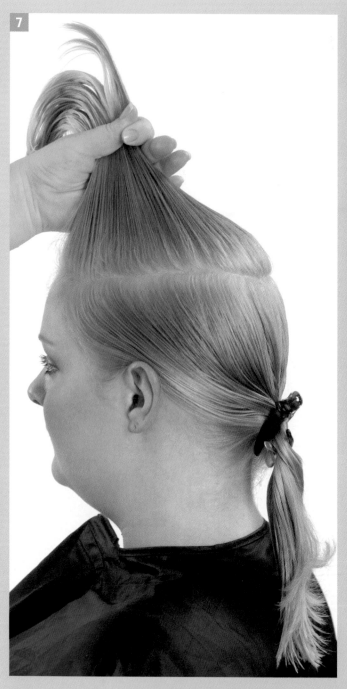

⑥ **Do this on both sides of the head right up to the centre parting, checking both sides are the same length after each cut. Once finished, re-check the length by combing all the hair back behind the ears and straight down at the back.**

⑦ **Re-part the hair down the centre from front to nape. Separate a section by parting from the hairline to the crown in a circular shape on both sides. Comb the rest of the hair from the sides and back to a bunch at the back and clip securely out of the way.**

**8**

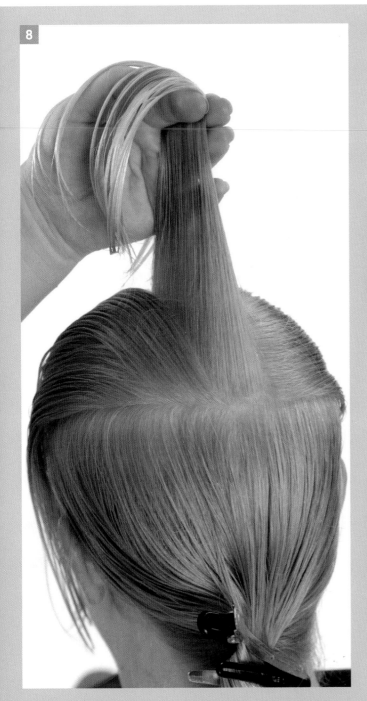

⑧ **Comb all the top section forward onto the face and take sections from the crown to the front hairline about 1–2 cm (0.5–1 in) thick.**

**9**

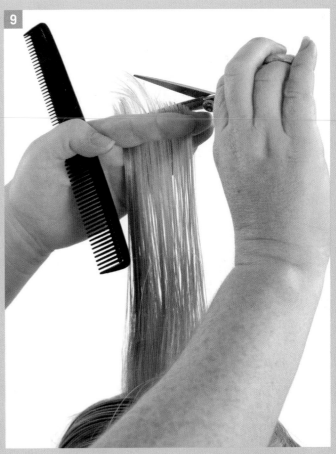

⑨ **Hold up the section at an angle, sloping down towards the face, and cut the amount of hair wanted to create the layer. This can be done either by chipping softly or club cutting in a straight line (which makes it easier to see the guideline). Work the whole of the top section in this way, holding the hair up straight and sloping down towards the face so that the hair is shorter around the face area.**

## tip

The angle of cut you decide on determines how short the hair is at the front and also how disconnected the cut is. The more slanted towards the front you cut, the shorter and more disconnected the end result will be; the less slanted towards the face you cut, the longer and less disconnected the layers.

▷

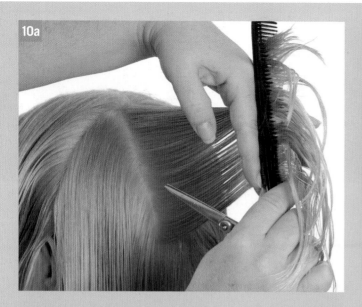

10a

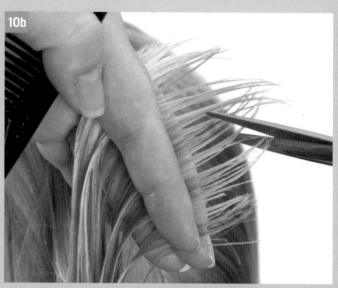

10b

⑩ab Once the top section is finished, comb it forward and let down the back hair. Take vertical sections and comb them out from the back of the head, chipping into the ends where needed to create layers.

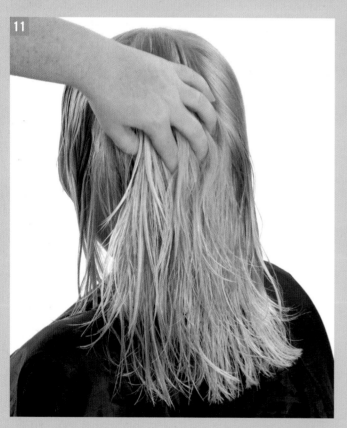

11

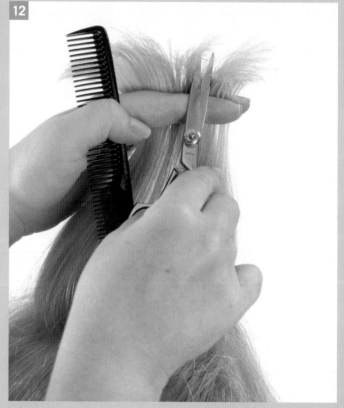

12

⑪ Run your hands through the hair and shake it out, making sure that you are happy with the layers created and the length you have taken out.

⑫ Dry the hair, then personalize according to the shape wanted by slicing or channel cutting out bulk, heavy areas or weight lines in the disconnection.

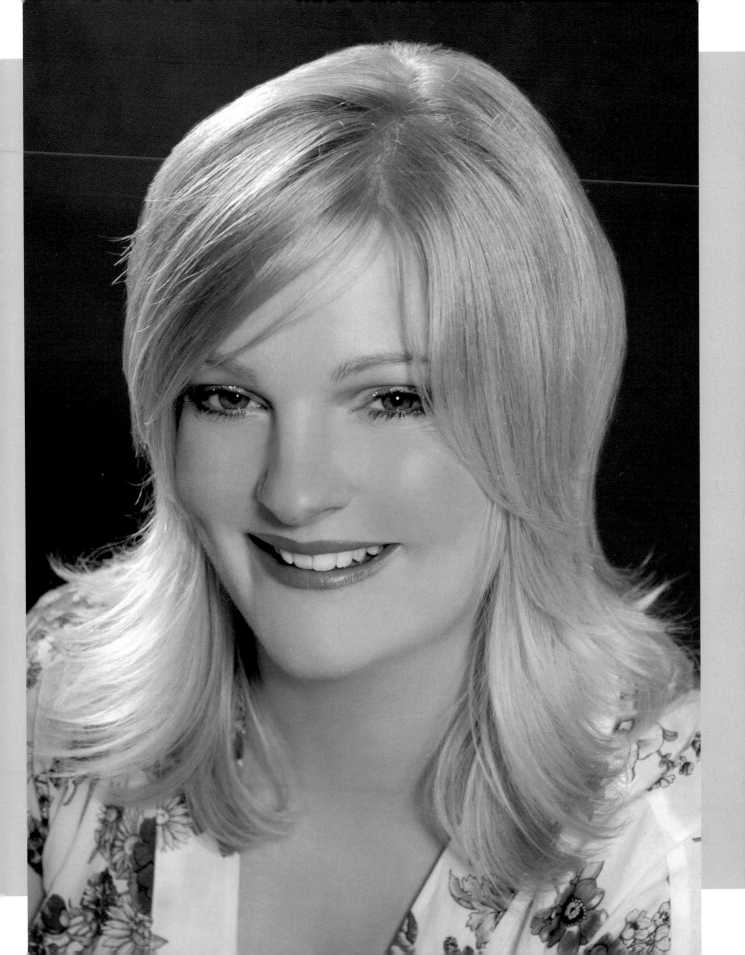

# cut personalizing

Personalizing a cut is often done when hair is dried into shape after the initial cut. It is a way of making the cut individual to each person according to their face shape and hair type, and also a way of creating your own personal, signature haircut. Personalizing creates extra softness or movement in a cut and can help to remove excess weight, blend in weight lines and remove bulk, which can make a huge difference as to how the hair lies. A stylist should, after blow-drying a cut, be able to see with the naked eye where there is weight or where the hair may need bulk removing from it; they should also be able to see where some softness of slices and texture may need adding to create a beautiful style.

Short hair, both men's and women's, can often need a lot more personalizing than other cuts, as weight lines or distribution of hair are more defined already due to the shortness of the hair. It also requires great care, as you do not want to keep cutting and cutting until there is no hair left – it has to be executed well!

Here is a guide to how each personalizing cut is done, but as with many skills in hairdressing, it takes a lot of practice to get it right and to become faster.

## Chipping

This can be used in both regular cutting when wet or personalizing when dry. It softens the edges of hair better than cutting in straight lines and can help to eliminate weight lines either used on its own or as part of the scissor over comb technique.

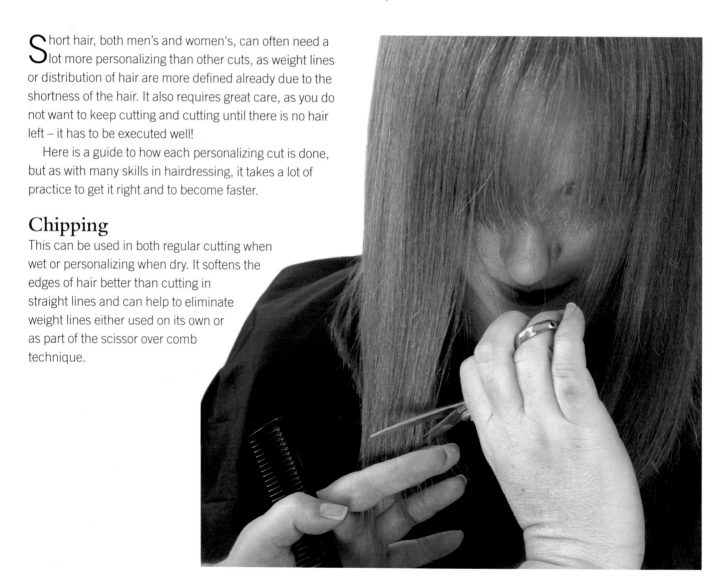

## Slicing

Slicing helps to soften a cut by creating texture and removing weight. It can remove a lot of excess bulk if hair is thick, creating shape whilst doing so. It is done by sliding the scissors through the mid-lengths to the ends of hair in very small pieces, removing excess unwanted hair. It can be used just on the ends if needed. If used too close to the roots it can leave small tufts of hair, so be careful – this technique is for mid-lengths and ends only.

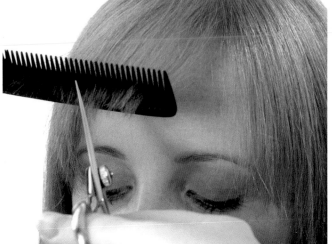

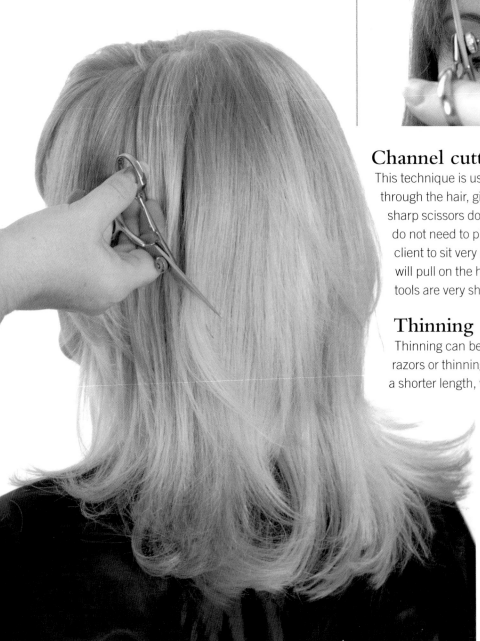

## Channel cutting

This technique is used to remove weight and create slices through the hair, giving texture. It is done by sliding very sharp scissors down the hair as it lies on the head – you do not need to pick the hair up, but it does require the client to sit very still. If your scissors are not sharp, they will pull on the hair and hurt the client, so mak sure your tools are very sharp.

## Thinning

Thinning can be done in any of the above ways or with razors or thinning scissors. It cuts small pieces of hair to a shorter length, which among the original hair length makes it appear thinner, but of course it is not permanent. You need to take extreme precaution when thinning hair not to cut and cut and cut, as you can remove too much and leave the hair looking extremely wispy and with no shape.

Thinning scissors remove the hair in a straight line, whereas slicing, chipping or channel cutting can be done in very small areas where needed. It is also done at different lengths to stop weight lines appearing, so is generally a more versatile approach.

# colouring hair: consultation

Colouring a client's hair can challenge even the best hairdresser. The result you achieve depends heavily on what condition the hair is in, so before looking deeper into colour you need to find out all about your client and their hair. This can be a time-consuming business, but it needs to be done thoroughly for the best results. Below are four areas that your consultation skills should be based around in order to get all the information you need.

## History

- Find out everything you can regarding what chemicals your client already has on their hair (this could be anything from perms and relaxers to colours, both permanent and temporary).

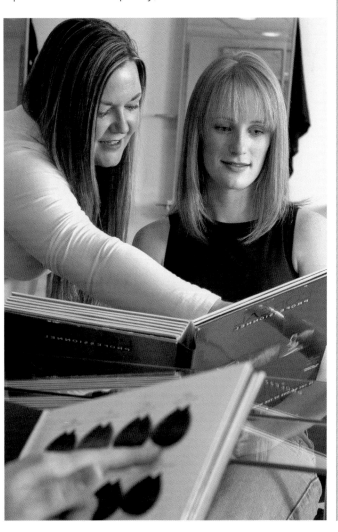

| tip |
| --- |

Remember that every inch of hair is around 2–4 months old depending on the speed of growth. So if the hair is long, it could be 3–4 years old at the ends, which means that even chemical treatments done long ago could affect the outcome. At the same time, just because someone's colour on the ends looks the same as the roots, it doesn't mean that all the hair has been treated the same all over. Always get a thorough history before you start.

- It is very important to find out if clients have had any reactions to chemical treatments in the past, as this could indicate that they are allergic to some of the chemicals used in colouring or perming. Be very cautious about applying or re-applying anything, and you should always do a skin test first.

## Lifestyle

- It is very useful to know a little bit about a client's lifestyle. For instance, what someone does for a living can help you to determine how soft or loud a colour should be. Giving a lawyer bright red hair and pink highlights is probably not advisable! Do they play sports? This can often mean that the hair is washed once a day or more, which could result in a colour fading more quickly. This will also help you to decide which type of colouring product to use.

- Lifestyle also affects maintenance, as you need to find out how often they are able to get their hair done. Many people

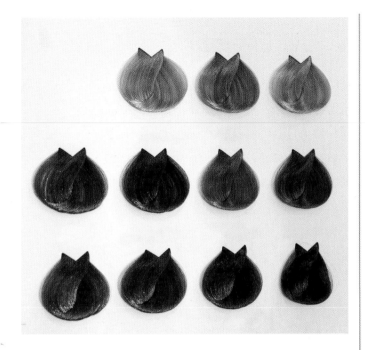

• Time is also a maintenance issue. How long can the client sit in the salon for and how often? If a client only has one hour to spare, you limit yourself to certain colouring products and applications as the time will not allow for longer and top-up colouring jobs.

• What products will your client be using at home? And will it help to prolong the beautiful colour she has just spent all that money and time on having done? Home-care is a must after colouring, and a good stylist should always recommend a suitable aftercare product – not for commission alone, but from a professional point of view. You have just spent one to two hours colouring your client's hair, and both for the client to make her colour and money last longer and also to ensure that the client does not return in a week saying her colour has faded, you should advise on the appropriate aftercare.

• Learning about a client's lifestyle also helps with maintenance advice – for instance, if a client swims they need to be aware that colour fades much more quickly with chlorine unless you protect it while in the pool. Blonde is not a great colour for heavy swimmers, as it has a tendency to turn green due to the chemicals used in pools. Brown hair might be a better option in this case.

are just too busy to get their colour done every four to six weeks, so this might help you to select colours that are suitable and will not look horrible with re-growth after four weeks. It will also affect the application of colour and your choice of method.

## Visuals

• Use as many visuals as possible for colouring – anything from official colour shade books to magazines, old photos and actual objects around you. This can help establish your idea of a colour compared to the client's. You'd be surprised how often they differ! Using a visual connects you and your client to the same colour and will help to achieve the right outcome.

## Maintenance

• This is a large area to cover and can involve questioning from all angles, from affordability to home care. You need to find out in a subtle way how much your client can afford to spend, and how often. This will help when choosing your colour and application method, as different applications differ in cost. It will also determine which colour type to use – if a client can only afford to have the colour re-done every ten weeks, then applying a full-head tint of permanent colour is not a good idea as the re-growth would be showing by then. Similarly, a full head of foil highlights are no good as this process is quite long and can be costly.

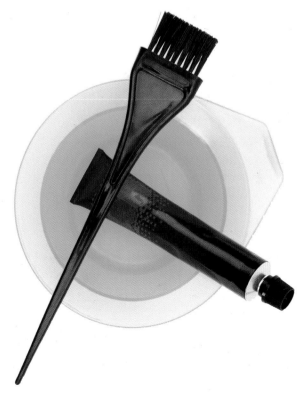

# types of colours

Colouring has expanded hugely over the last 10–15 years and has become a large money-making business in hair salons everywhere. It requires skill and knowledge to use it correctly and can result in major problems if not used appropriately. To make your life easier, in the professional colouring industry there is something called an ICC, or International Colour Code. This enables you to use any colouring product from a listed company knowing that their system of colouring numbers and codes should be similar.

Whether you buy colour from a supermarket or use it professionally, it is very important even if you are highly trained to follow each individual manufacturer's instructions, as they can differ from company to company. Manufacturers go to a lot of trouble testing colours and instructing you on how to use them to get the correct results, so it makes sense to listen to their advice.

Colours generally come in five categories:

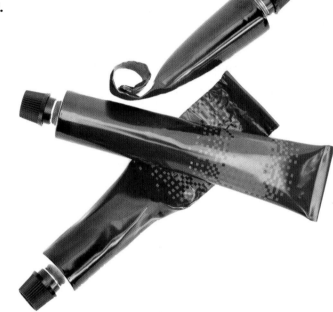

## Temporary

These normally come in a mousse or setting lotion form, but are also now available in sprays. They usually add tones to white hair, for instance (such as pearl or honey-coloured tones), but they would not cover white hair completely. You don't have to mix them – they are applied straight out of their container – and they only last until the hair is washed again.

## Semi-permanent

Normally these are lotions or come in a shampoo form and are never mixed with anything – you use them directly out of their applicator bottle or sachet. They last on average about 6–8 washes but this depends on the hair's history and whether it already has chemicals on it, as this can cause the colour to last longer. They can only make the hair darker or stay the same colour, but can also add tones such as reds, coppers and golds.

## Quasi colour

These usually come in a gel, lotion or cream form but are mixed with a low oxidant or an activator in most cases. They gradually fade from the hair as opposed to being washed out

or grown out, and last from 6–8 weeks. Quasi colours are in between semi and permanent colours and are known by some people as demi colours. They cannot lighten hair but can make it go darker or stay the same, adding vibrant tones such as reds, coppers, gold or ashes.

---

### tip

**FOR QUASI COLOUR**

People sometimes unwittingly buy quasi colours from chemists or grocery stores, telling you when they come to the salon that they have used a semi colour. Be aware that this can affect colouring in the salon, as they have an oxidant base.

---

## Permanent

Normally always in cream or liquid form and always mixed with an oxidant of 20 volume (6 per cent) or above. This colour will permanently change the hair structure and colour and will either grow out or be cut out. Permanent colours can make hair lighter, darker, cover white completely, add strong tones to the existing hair colour, or change the tones completely.

## Bleach

Normally a powder or cream-type paste and always mixed with an oxidant of 20 volume (6 per cent) or above. This product removes natural pigment from the hair and any other colouring products, unless the hair is particularly dense. It permanently changes the hair colour and can only be cut or grown out. It always makes the hair go lighter but not necessarily evenly, so be careful when using it. Bleach can be found in chemists and grocery stores but only to certain strengths – salons can use a stronger solution of bleach as the staff will be professionally trained to do so.

## How do they work?

- **Temporary colour** sits on the cuticle and only lasts one shampoo.
- **Semi-permanent colour** penetrates a little deeper into the cuticle and lasts for 6–8 washes.
- **Quasi colour** sits just inside the cortex and in the cuticle and fades gradually over an average of 8–12 washes, depending on the manufacturer
- **Permanent colour/bleach** goes into the cortex and physically changes the hair's natural pigments and only grows out or is cut out.

## HAIR STRUCTURE

To understand colour you need to understand a little about the hair's structure. The main thing to understand when it comes to colour is that the hair has three layers: the cuticle, or outside layer; the cortex, or inside layer; and the medulla, or centre. See the 'How do they work?' feature to the left to understand where the different colours sit.

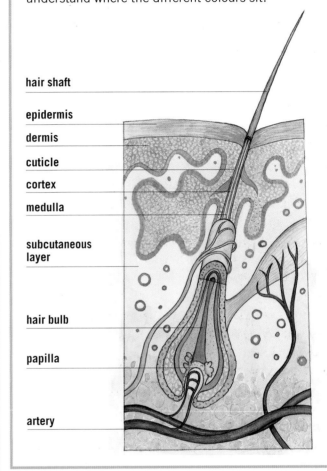

- hair shaft
- epidermis
- dermis
- cuticle
- cortex
- medulla
- subcutaneous layer
- hair bulb
- papilla
- artery

# natural colours of hair

Inside the human hair there are two natural pigments that determine your natural hair colour. These are melanin and pheomelanin. Melanin appears in brownish-black colours and makes up the majority of your base colour or the depth – how light or dark you are – whereas pheomelanin appears in reddish-yellow colours and makes up the tones you have in your hair which sometimes you see and sometimes you don't.

Redheads have a lot of pheomelanin in their hair, hence the appearance of red or copper colours. Asian hair has a lot too, but because of the density and amount of melanin in the hair you cannot see it. If you were to put bleach on the hair, the first colours that would appear would be red/orange/yellow, and often you will not be able to reach a very light blonde or white colour on Asian hair.

Afro hair has a lot of melanin pigment but not much

pheomelanin, so when bleached it can lift to blonde very easily. However, the hair structure is often fragile so may not withstand too much bleaching or heavy colouring.

To understand colour even more, we need to go back to our primary colours of red, yellow and blue. If you mix all three you get brown, and depending on the quantities of each that you use, you can get all the different shades of natural hair from black through to very light blonde, which is

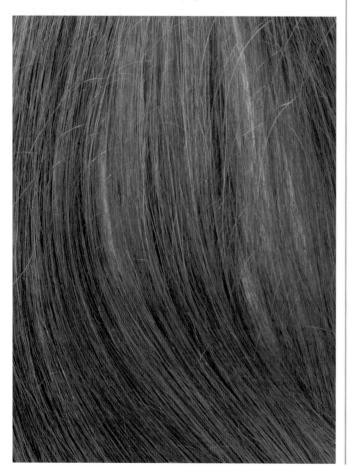

technically speaking the melanin pigment. The pheomelanin is just two of the colours – red and yellow – which can appear orange.

All hair has an 'undercoat' colour, and most colour manufacturers produce a chart to help you gauge what colour that undercoat is. When you apply any type of oxidant or peroxide to hair, the undercoat will lighten according to the strength of the oxidant. If the undercoat is too light for a colour, the colour will fade more quickly; if the undercoat is too warm for the colour required, it will affect the end result of the colour chosen. As a rough guide, you will often find that the darker the natural colour of the hair (e.g. black), the darker the undercoat (red, in this case).

Undercoats are normally always red, orange or yellow, with red being the more dominant colour (being the strongest undercoat) and yellow the least. It is important that you consider the undercoat when choosing a colour, as it can affect the end results. Another important factor to remember is that some colours neutralize others out, and a colour wheel will help you to identify which neutralizes which. If someone has brown hair with red tones that you wish to get rid of, or neutralize, the opposite colour in the colour wheel will do so. You could therefore put on a brown

## THE COLOUR WHEEL

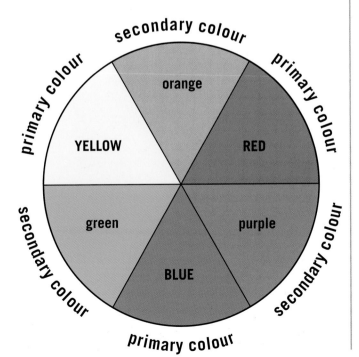

## HAIR COLOURS AND NUMBERING SYSTEMS

According to the ICC (International Colour Code), numbering for natural hair colours such as brown, blonde and black run on a scale of 1 to 10. The following colours have their undercoats in brackets.

1 = black (red)
2 = darkest brown (red)
3 = dark brown (red)
4 = brown (red)
5 = light brown (red/orange)
6 = dark blonde (orange)
7 = blonde (yellow/orange)
8 = light blonde (yellow)
9 = very light blonde (pale yellow)
10 = lightest blonde (very pale yellow)

colour with green tones and it would eliminate (neutralize) the red. If you have orange tones, adding blue to a colour would neutralize the orange and so on. Putting blue into a colour may sound drastic, but always remember that hair colours are not like other colours. Blue in this case might just be an ash colour tinged with blue.

## Tones

Tones are also made from the primary colours – in fact, the primary colours alone are tones – but if mixed together:

**Red** and **yellow** = **orange**
**Red** and **blue** = **mauve/violet ash**
**Yellow** and **blue** = **green**

Some colours have one tone and some two, but rarely are there more than this. They are also given numbers, names or letters to identify them:

**Red** is often a 6 or the letter R
**Coppers** are a 4 or letter K
**Gold** is a 3 or letter G
**Mauve/violet ash** is a 5 or possibly a letter such as A
**Blue ash** is a 1 or possibly a letter such as B

You should always identify each one separately according to the manufacturer.

# oxidants

In salons you can find oxidants from 20 volume (6 per cent) to 40 volume (12 per cent) and even sometimes 60 volume (18 per cent), which is very rarely used nowadays as the products are so good that you don't need such strong oxidants.

You will need to know the outcome of using different oxidants. A general scale for use is as follows:

### 20 volume (6 per cent)
- To lift hair one or two shades lighter than natural base.
- To cover white hair.
- To keep hair the same base colour but change tone.
- To go darker.
- Lifts undercoat two levels from natural colour.

### 30 volume (9 per cent)
- To lift hair three shades lighter than natural base.
- Lifts undercoat three levels from natural base.

### 40 volume (12 per cent)
- To lift hair four shades lighter than natural base.
- Must not be used on scalp – only for foil or partial techniques.
- Lifts undercoat four levels from natural base.

Finding out a product's strengths is very important, and you need to research every different product that you use. Some products will lighten hair to a different degree and their development time and mixtures all vary, so it is imperative to find this out and then use the rules of general oxidant power with the appropriate product.

# selecting your colour

Firstly do a step-by-step analysis of the colour of your client's hair. Look at the natural base and tones – whether natural or old colour. Remember to use the consultation guide to get a good understanding of the hair's colour history.

## tip

Remember to note all colour analysis on record cards. Look at the colour on the lengths and ends of the hair, as the end of the hair may be a different colour to the roots. Are the base and tones natural? What colour are the lengths, ends and tones?

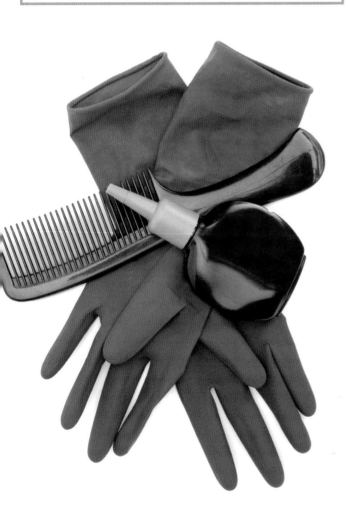

After completing the consultation you should have a good idea of which type of colour to use – semi or permanent, etc. – and after consultation you should have a good idea of how much colour to use, be it full head or partial. Now you need to decide on the actual colour. Is the client going lighter, staying same or going darker than the natural colour? For example, if you have analyzed the natural base to be 6 (dark blonde) and the client wishes to be a brown, it is going darker. If she is a 6 and wishes to be an 8, it is going lighter. This would be going lighter by two levels, which indicates that you should use 20 volume or 6 per cent, and that your undercoat would also go from a 6 to an 8. A typical equation, therefore, would look like this:

**NB** 6
**L&E** ?
**SR** 8
**LL 2** = 20 VOLUME OXIDANT 6%
**UC** Y = 8

**KEY:**
**NB** = Natural base colour (6 in this case).
**L&E** = Lengths and ends colour (none in this case, hence the question mark).
**SR** = Shade required by client (8 in this case).
**LL** = How many levels of lightening are required? (The answer – two in this case – will determine which oxidant peroxide you choose. 20 volume oxidant lifts the shade two levels, as required.)
**UC** = Undercoat that will appear when using an oxidant (Y, or yellow, in this case – according to the shade chart on page 81, which makes the outcome an 8, which is what the client wants).

Is the tone that is already present in their hair compatible with the tone they want? If a base 8 is the shade required (which is light blonde), the undercoat is yellow which will show through and the client will end up with a warm base 8 result. So you need to eliminate the impact of the undercoat by neutralizing and using a 8 with mauve ash. This will give client a perfect result of a light blond 8. If the tones are compatable, then you will be able to apply the colour in whichever technique you have chosen without neutralizing.

## GREEN HAIR

Green hair tends to affect bleached or light-coloured hair. It is never seen in black hair, as the green gets lost in the background colour. It can often be seen in regular swimmers, and can also be caused by traces of copper in water. Green hair can even appear after a good long soak in a bath that has been cleaned with bathroom cleaners containing high chloride levels. Occasionally it can simply be the result of using bleach. There are soft cleansing products available that help to remove the green tinge. Any green must be removed from hair before colouring as it can alter the appearance of any subsequent colour you use.

## COVERING WHITE HAIR

Most companies create a base range of colours numbered 1–10. They have to be added to all other colours to cover white hair, as using permanent colours that are 'fashion shades' alone will not cover white. You will often need to apply large quantities of the base colour, as the hair absorbs a lot. Development times vary according to each manufacturer, but some will extend the time by few minutes or to full maximum timing for proper white coverage.

## tip

Remember that colour does not lift already-present colour, so if a client wants to go lighter and already has colour on their hair it will require bleaching out or colour correction first, which is a technique for very advanced hairdressers only.

## trade secrets and tips

### FOR COLOUR

- Remember when applying dark colours to hair to apply a barrier cream around the hairline and on the tops of ears before you start. This will prevent the client from getting a stain on forehead or ears.

- Don't be misled by a colour's appearance when on the hair, as it often does not resemble the colour of the finished (dry) hair.

- Always follow the manifacturer's instructions for timing on colour application. Taking the colour off early will only make the colour fade more quickly – it will not

make it a softer or lighter colour. Nor will removing it much later than the recommended time make the colour last longer – in fact it will do the opposite as it will damage the hair's internal structure, making it harder for the colour to take and making it fade more quickly.

- Advise the client to use colour-enhancing conditioners as the colour grows out, to help blend the root areas with the rest of the hair.

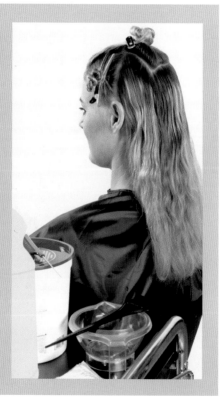

# sectioning for colour

Sectioning hair is important in all areas of hairdressing, but it is particularly important when colouring hair. It makes the whole process less messy and also makes it easier to apply the colour in a methodical way.

### Nine section
This sectioning pattern would be used for a full head of highlights, allowing it to follow a neat application pattern.

### Half head sectioning pattern
Used to highlight half a head only in a neat pattern.

### Partial or T-section
Used to do partial highlights on mainly the top of the head, and sometimes the sides as well.

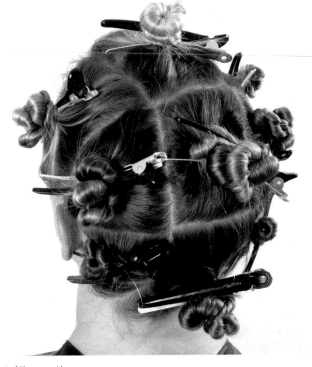

△ Nine section

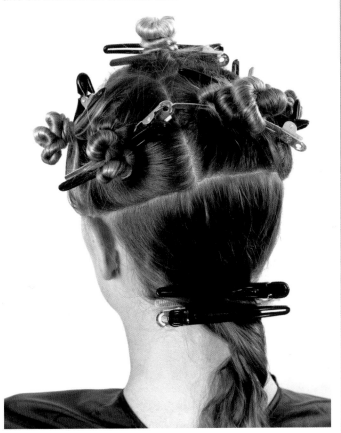

△ Half head section

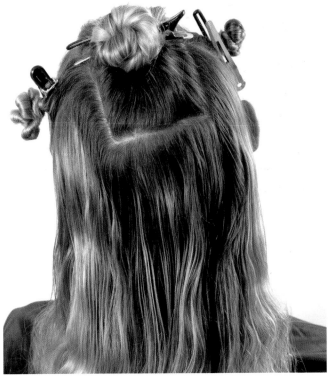

△ Partial/T-section

# semi/quasi/permanent tint

The application method is the same for all of these tints. Always have a trolley prepared ready and close beside you for use during colouring, and wear gloves and an apron for protection.

## how to...

### APPLY SEMI, QUASI OR PERMANENT TINTS

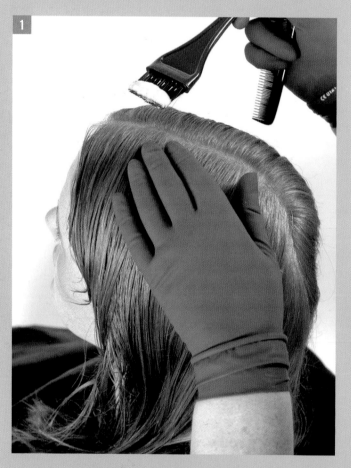

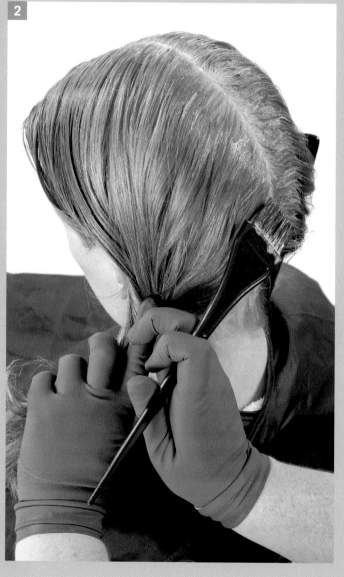

① Part hair from front to nape down the middle and paste the colour on, starting at the front on the root area of the hair and covering around 2.5 cm (1 in).

② Work through the whole parting, pasting colour on both sides of the part from front to nape.

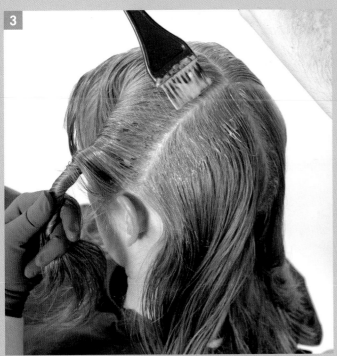

③ Part the hair from the crown to the ear on one side and paste colour on both sides of the parting on the root area.

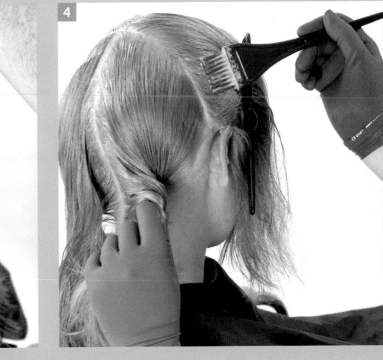

④ Do the same to the other side. You should have four sections clearly visible and separated.

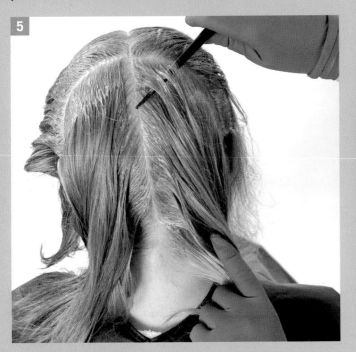

⑤ Starting at the back sections, take one section and, near the crown, using the end of a tail comb, take a sub-section across about 1 cm (0.5 in) thick.

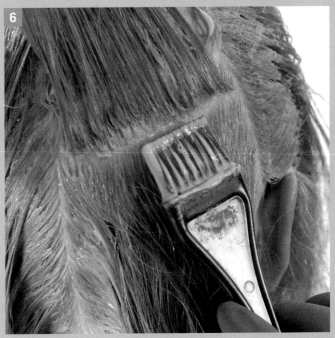

⑥ Hold this section up and paste colour on both sides of the sub-section at the root. Lay the section up and over the top of the head.

▷

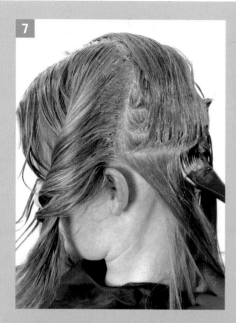

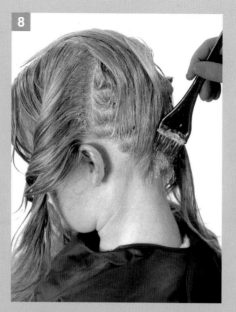

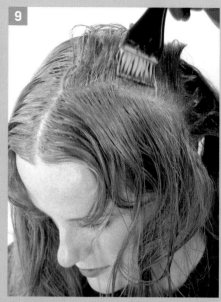

⑦ Take another sub-section across just below the last one, again 1 cm (0.5 in) thick. Working at this thickness should allow you to see the colour seep through from the other side where the last colour was pasted. If not, take thinner sections to avoid missing areas.

⑧ Paste colour on either side of the section's roots and continue in this way right down to the nape. Once completed, lightly pick up the ends of the sections coloured and pull them back over to lie on top of the section they have been taken from.

⑨ Move to the next section at the back of the head and repeat the process. For the front sections, if the sub-sections become too wide, take slightly smaller sub-sections with less width and keep the sections thin enough to see the colour pasted on the last one.

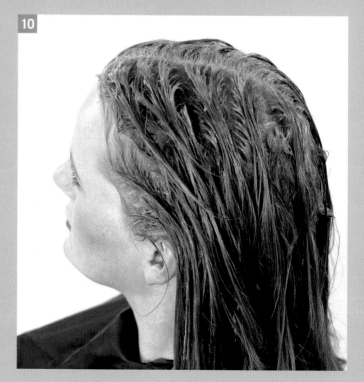

⑩ Once done, develop according to the manufacturer's instructions. The lengths and ends can also be coloured if wanted.

# lengths and ends application

These are general guidelines for lengths and ends application, but it is best to consult the manufacturer's instructions and apply according to their recommendations.

## how to...

### COLOUR THE LENGTHS AND ENDS

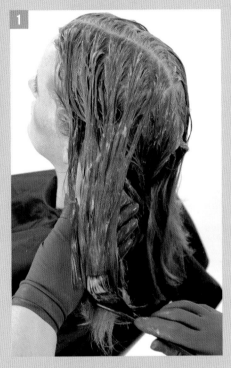

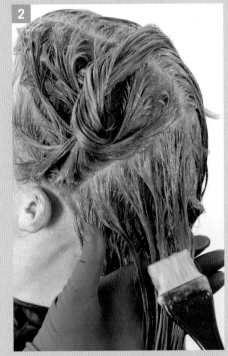

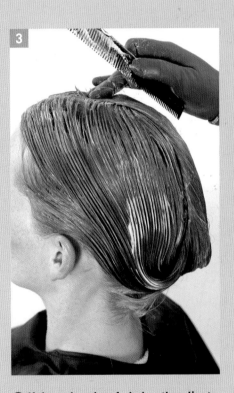

① If the client is staying the same colour as usual, and the colour is still the same on the ends and has not faded, you just need to emulsify the mixture. Apply the colour to the roots, develop fully, then just add a little water and brush onto the ends for a few minutes.

② If the colour is the same but has faded slightly from sun, chlorine or any other reason, you need to add a little more colour. Take the colour through by applying to the roots, develop for half the manufacturer's recommended development time, then add about 10–20 mls of water to about a quarter of a tube of remaining tint mix. Apply to the lengths and ends, then develop for the rest of the manufacturer's recommended development time.

③ If the colour has faded or the client is changing the colour to something similar to before, you need to take through all the colour in one go. Apply the colour to the roots, then add 10–20 mls of water to the remaining quarter of a tube of colour mixture. Apply to lengths and ends immediately, comb through, then develop according to the instructions. If the client wants a lighter shade, an advanced colouring assessment will be needed.

# full-head colouring

Unlike a regular tint application, this is done the other way around, with the lengths and ends coloured first. This is because, often, the hair has never been coloured before, and the ends tend to be harder to colour than the roots.

## how to...

### APPLY FULL-HEAD COLOUR

Before mixing and applying colour to all lengths and ends, first separate the hair into sections as you would for a regular tint application.

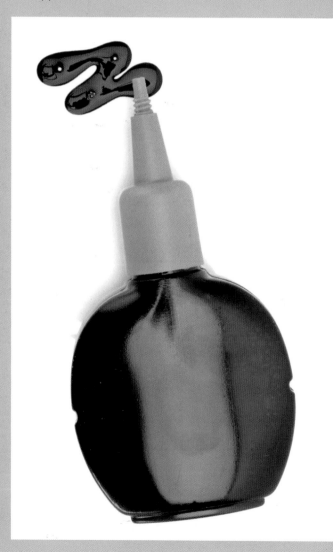

① Part the hair from front to nape, then add the colour. Part the hair from ear to ear and add colour as before to lengths and ends. Starting at the back, take sub-sections across from the nape up and apply colour to the mid-lengths and ends leaving only 2.5 cm (1 in) at the roots un-coloured. Allow it to develop for half of the recommended development time.

② Mix up the same colour but fresh, and then apply to the roots and overlap to the ends again, without adding water. Once applied to the roots, allow to develop for the full recommended time.

③ Shampoo and style as usual.

# shoe-shine colour

This technique can be used for both men's hair and women's short hair to add colour. It can be applied just to the top or all over to create a soft, natural, sunkissed look, or a stronger look if more colour is applied.

## how to...

**APPLY SHOE-SHINE COLOUR**

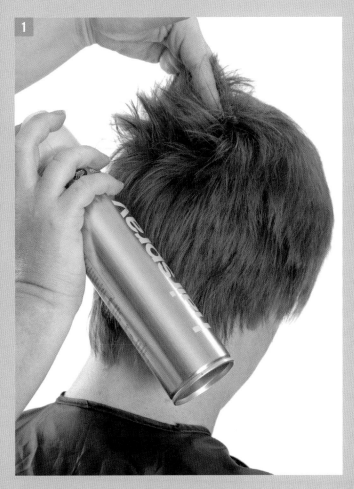

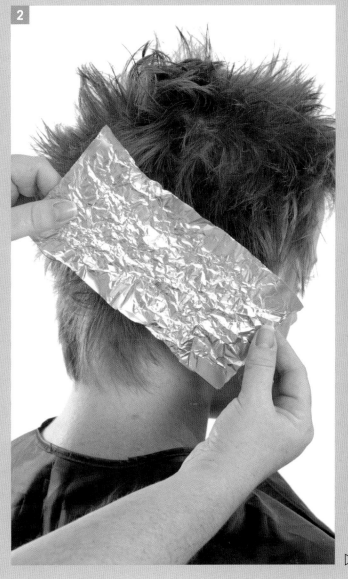

① Dry the hair spiky, and spray with hairspray to make it stand up even straighter. This will make the application neater.

② Take a piece of foil, scrunch it up carefully without ripping it and then open it back up.

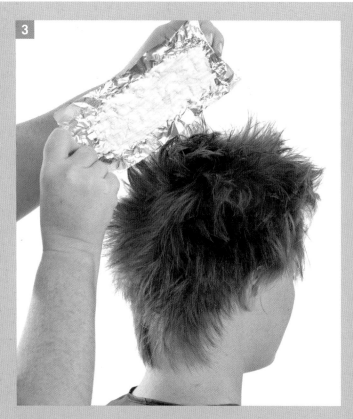

③ Brush pre-mixed bleach or prelightener onto it.

④ Brush it over the ends of the hair as if you are shining shoes. Do this all over the hair and on the back as well, if long enough.

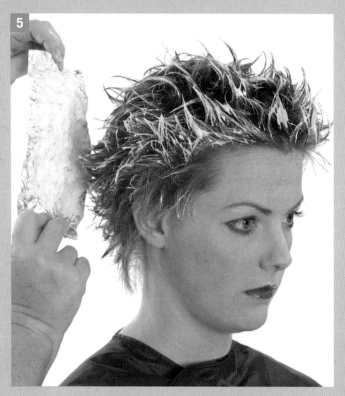

⑤ Allow it to develop to the required colour, and if needed add heat to speed the process up. Shampoo off and style.

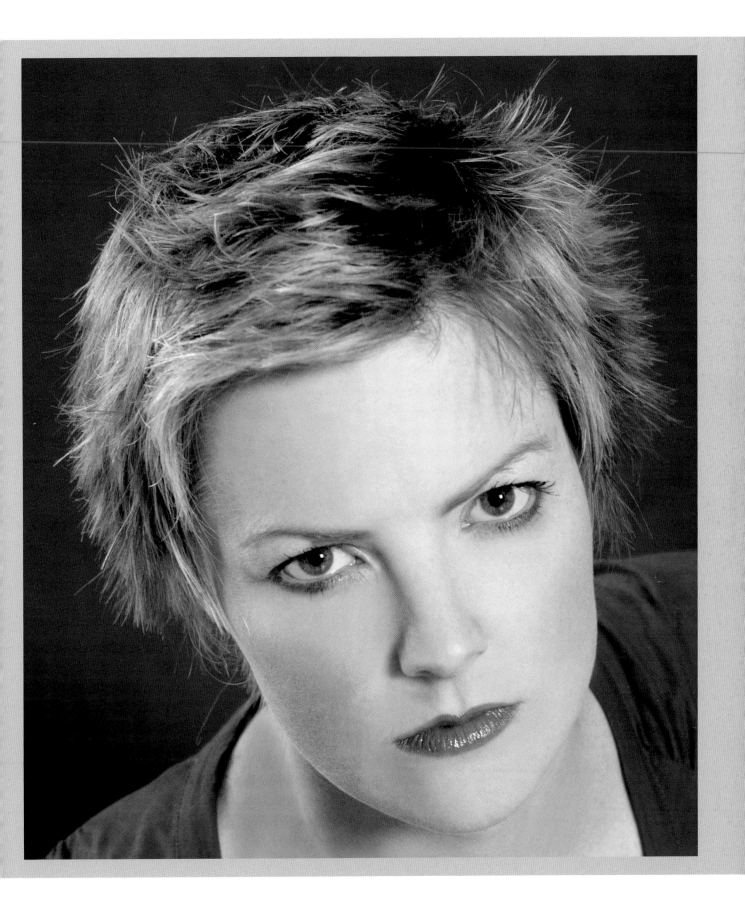

# alternatives to shoe-shine colour

## SMUDGE COLOUR

This is an alternative colouring method to the shoe-shine technique for short hair. Follow the method for length and ends application using a semi, quasi or permanent tint and take through to the roots, but leave out odd bits of the ends from the colour. Pre-mix some bleach and scrunch into the ends without the colour, then develop according to the manufacturer's instructions.

## PAINT-ON COLOUR

Another alternative, this look creates soft flashes of colour over the hair in the areas you want it to appear. After cutting hair and combing into shape, select the colour required by using the guide to colour selection, although this technique works better with bleach. Using a tint brush on its side, paint fine individual lines of colour onto the hair. Do not put too close together, and only do fine lines and not too many. Develop with no heat.

## FLOODLIGHTS

Apply full-colour tint, although if it is for a man, chose a flat colour, preferably without red or yellow tones, for the best result. Once applied, mix up a small amount of bleach with 30 volume oxidant. As with the paint-on technique, paint lines over the colour already on the hair. The lines of bleach can be thicker this time as they create a soft 'floodlight' effect, as if the hair is shining in those areas. The colour chosen for the base colour must be a dark or deeper colour for floodlights to show effectively.

## tip

### FOR SMUDGE COLOUR

This can be a rather messy application but the colour turns out extremely well. On men it is good to select a flat colour for the root application of the semi/quasi tint so that it looks natural.

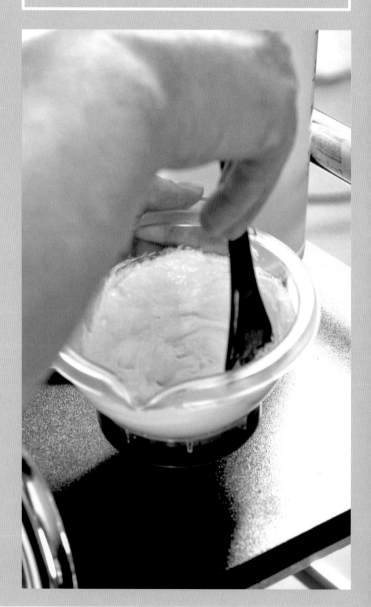

# foils application

Hairdressers apply foils in many ways, depending on how they feel comfortable doing it. This method works for me, and always bear in mind that the more practice you get, the better you will become.

## how to...

### APPLY FOILS FOR HIGHLIGHTS

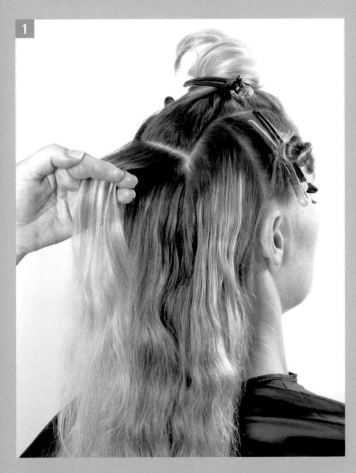

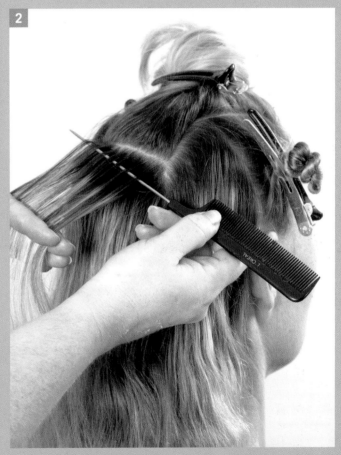

① Separate hair into a sectioning pattern according to the amount of highlights to be done. Start at the first section and take a sub-section across no thicker than 0.5 cm (0.25 in) or thinner, according to the size of highlight required.

② Weave pieces of hair from the section. Your weave depends on the thickness of the highlight required – the thicker the weave, the thicker the highlight. However it also depends on hair density – if the hair is thick, a fine highlight may not show up, so judge according to hair density and the required result.

▷

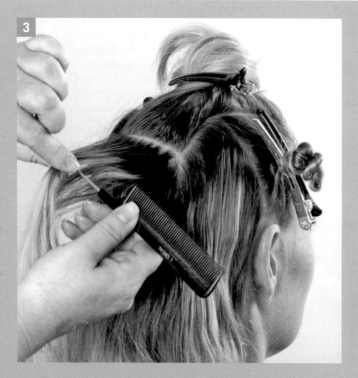

③ Separate the weaved pieces from the rest of the section and hold the weaves taut.

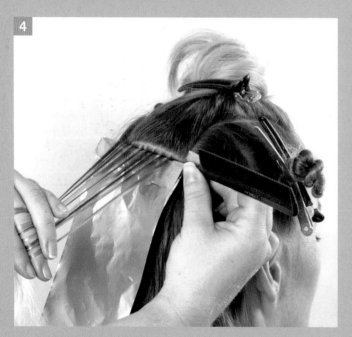

④ Keep hold of the comb and pick up one foil. Place the foil into the root by folding the foil around the tail comb and pushing it into the root area underneath the section you are holding.

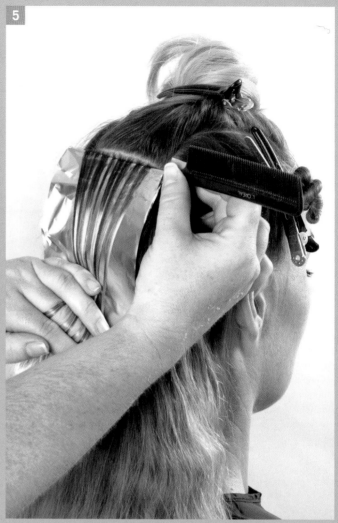

⑤ Once it is in the right position, hold the hair down over the foil very tightly, helping to hold the foil in place. Remove the tail comb carefully.

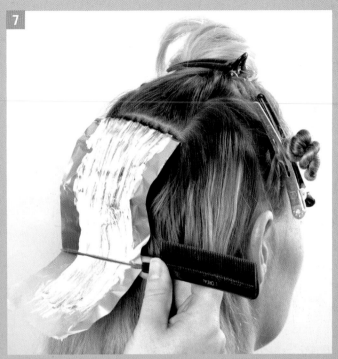

⑦ Without pulling on the foil, gently use the tail comb to indent a fold almost halfway up and fold the foil in half.

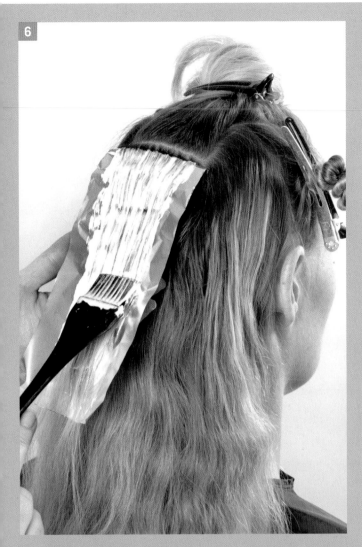

⑥ Apply some colour to the tint brush. Don't apply too much, but don't skimp on on it or you will move the foil as the tint brush has no product on it. Apply the colour about 2 cm (1 in) away from the root, then slowly apply up to the edge.

## tip

Don't go too close to the edge or you will get bleed marks, or seepage of the colour out of the foil, which will spoil the results. Apply colour right down to the ends of the hair unless it is not needed – just to mid-lengths or roots only may be fine depending on how much re-growth there is.

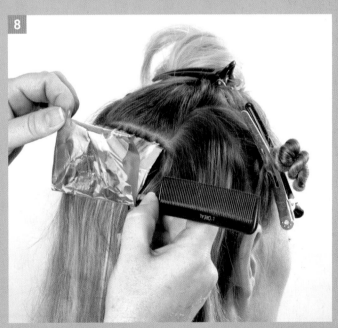

⑧ Fold in half again if needed, and try to line up the bottom edge with the top edge of the foil. Do not pat down or flatten the foil, as this can push colour out of the packet and create bleeding or seeping.

▷

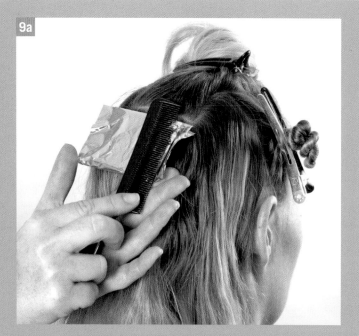

**9a**

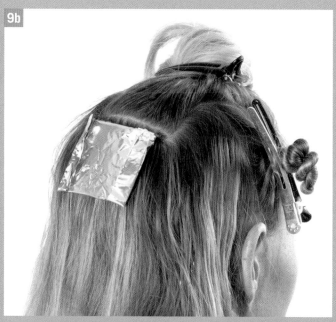

**9b**

⑨ab **Using the comb end of the tail comb, mark an indent on the edges of packet and fold in both sides of the foil just a**

couple of millimetres. **Again, don't flatten the packet or the colour will seep.**

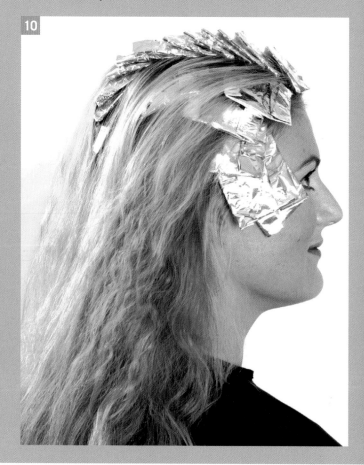

**10**

⑩ **Repeat this process in a neat and orderly fashion through the sections put in place, remembering to keep the weave and the sub-sections the same thickness throughout. Leave to develop as per the manufacturer's instructions before washing out and styling.**

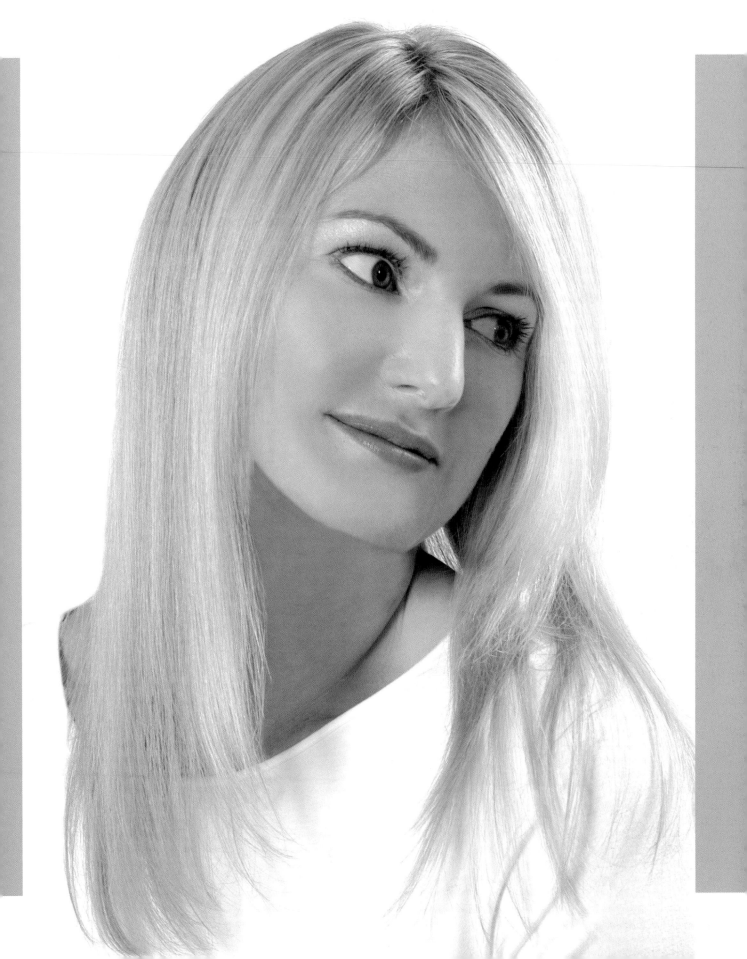

# the perm

People have been trying to to turn straight hair into waves and curls for thousands of years. Ancient Egyptian women used to apply a mixture of soil and water to their hair, wrap it on handmade wooden rollers and then bake the mud in the sun. The results would have been anything but permanent, but temporarily curling hair is still achieved by setting damp, wet or dry hair into a new shape on curlers, rollers or by using tongs. The changes to the hair are the same as Egyptian women would have experienced – only the weak bonds in the hair are affected, and the hair goes back to its original shape as soon as it is dampened again.

The first true perms, or permanent waves, became available in the early 1900s, when the perming lotion was activated by heat from an electrical device plugged into the ceiling. The early models did not have thermostats, and it was difficult to control their temperature. They had individual heaters for each curl, and clients found these heavy and uncomfortable. These early perms were harsh and drying, and left the hair in tight frizzy curls that were difficult to manage.

In the 1940s, the 'cold wave' was introduced. This was basically the perming process that we use today. The cold wave had many advantages: the unpleasant heat and weight of the old appliances were completely eliminated, and the hair could be waved closer to the scalp. Unfortunately, these days perming seems to have fallen out of fashion, and you will not be asked to do it very often except for some of the older generation who still like it done. Fashions change, however, and it is very important that you retain this skill. Understanding the chemistry behind it and what is actually happening to the hair is the first step.

## Hair bonds

There are many types of bonds inside the hair that are like chains or links that hold the structural

## HOW HAIR BONDS WORK

On the left you can see the normal internal chemical structure of the hair protein, showing unbroken disulphide bonds. The central diagram show what happens during perming, when bonds in the hair wrapped around a roller are broken by a perming lotion. On the right we see the hair as it looks after neutralizing – the bonds are rejoined and realigned in a different order, permanently changing the shape and producing a curl. This is how a perm is created.

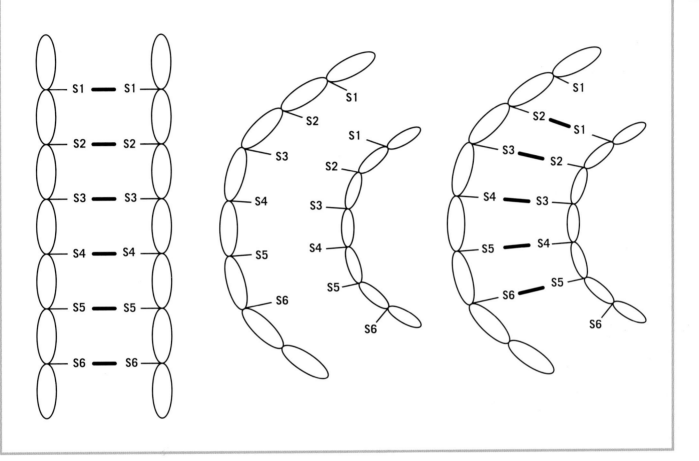

shape of the hair. Two of these are saline bonds and disulphide bonds.

Saline bonds are broken every time you wet your hair with water. Every time your hair dries, whether it is naturally, round a brush or even in rollers, they rejoin into the shape in which you dry your hair. So for instance, if one day you have straight hair then the next you shampoo it and set it on rollers, the shape will change and stay that way until the next time the hair is washed. This is achieved by breaking (wetting) and rejoining (drying) the bonds.

Disulphide bonds are different in only one way – they only break and rejoin with certain chemicals instead of water, and it is these chemicals that are found in perm lotions, relaxers and neutralizers.

The first stage of perm lotion breaks down the bonds when put onto hair that is in rollers, which is what creates the new shape. To rejoin them is slightly more complicated, as you need another chemical to rejoin the disulphide bond. This is called a neutralizer, a lotion that when applied rejoins the disulphide bonds back into the shape they are now in. If the hair is wound round a perm roller the bonds will make the hair curly, or if combed very straight they will straighten it. The bigger the roller the hair is wound around, the bigger the curl; the smaller the roller, the tighter the curl.

## Perm lotion

When first consulting a client, you have to decide which lotion type to use, as perm lotion comes in different strengths according to hair type. Hair only can absorb a certain amount of liquid, whether it be water or perm solution. The amount absorbed depends greatly on the hair texture, but often more coarse or resistant hair takes more liquid and weaker, sensitized hair takes less. Always bear in mind, however, that if the lotion is too strong for the hair, it could damage it further.

The different strengths of solution are for different hair types as follows:
- ★ **Natural resistant**
- ★ **Natural**
- ★ **Coloured**
- ★ **Coloured sensitized**

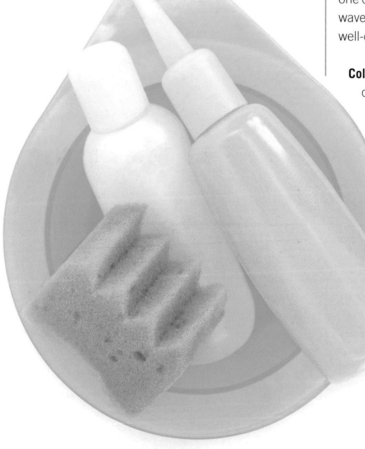

| tip |
| --- |

Never perm hair that is more than slightly damaged with colour, as this may result in serious hair damage and breakage.

The following guide should help you to identify which type to use.

**Natural resistant** hair is usually glossy and shiny. It is normally always naturally straight, or if it has a wave it is white or grey hair, possibly coarse in texture. When blow-dried it does not stay in shape for long and drops its shape very easily; when shampooing, water runs off the hair at first and takes a while to soak in.

**Natural** describes hair with only temporary or semi colour, one quasi colour or none at all. It can have a slight bend or wave, it holds its shape well with blow-dries and is generally well-controlled hair.

**Coloured** hair is any hair with two or more colours (be they quasi, permanent or bleached) but the hair is generally in good condition.

**Colour sensitized** is hair that has been repeatedly coloured and may be sensitized or slightly damaged.

## Rollers

Once you have determined the lotion to use, you need to decide on a suitable roller size. This depends to a large extent on hair length – if you put a large roller in short hair and the same roller in long hair, the size of curl will differ according to the amount of hair being wound around it. On short hair it would only give root lift and not much curl, as the hair would only just go round the roller, whereas with long hair it would give soft curls as the hair may go around the roller several times.

These days rollers come in many types – see page 19 for more information. Generally they all give curl, but some give a softer curl, some a more definite curl, and some are used just to give volume and movement.

Once you have selected the roller size, you need to decide on a wind technique. There are many of these, some of which are listed on pages 110–111. The size of the section you take to put each roller in has a great effect on the size of the curl, so be precise with this. A section size should normally be 1 cm (0.5 in) shorter than the length of the actual roller (if using regular rollers) and the width of the section should be slightly slimmer than the roller itself. If this is done correctly you will get the right curl size according to the roller size selected.

Some rollers, such as Molton Browners, or 'bendies' as some call them, take a little more hair per roller, but not much more. You will not get a good curl result if too much hair is put around a roller. Bendy rollers simply make it easier to perm long hair and to create spiral or corkscrew winds.

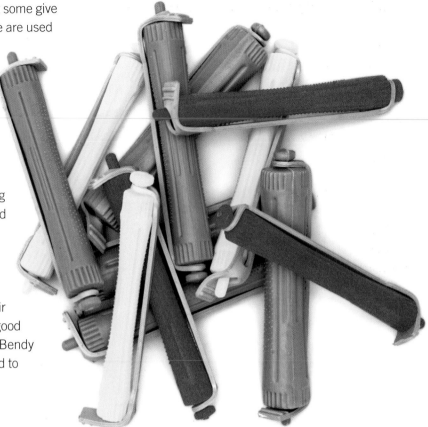

## trade secrets and tips

### FOR PERMING

- If the hair is bagging out from the side or looks loose when winding rollers for a set or perm, it means the section is too big for the roller. Take it out and make the section smaller with less hair.

- As the perm grows out, advise the client to spray a volumizing product or gel at the roots and blow-dry at the scalp to create added lift.

- Ensure that your client makes an appointment for a trim. It's important to get your hair trimmed every 5-6 weeks to remove the ends. Trimming will also extend the life of the perm and make it easier for the client to style.

- A perm will take better if the client has not washed their hair in the past 24 hours. Always advise your clients of this when you take their booking.

- Advise your client not to wrap their hair in a towel turban when they get out of the shower with wet hair. The friction can knot and damage vulnerable wet hair. Instead, carefully blot hair dry.

- Only brush or comb permed hair while it is wet, as brushing or combing when dry will make it look frizzy and bushy.

# Sectioning

The sectioning pattern of the rollers is the next important thing to decide. These are standard with all roller types and are either nine sections, brick or directional.

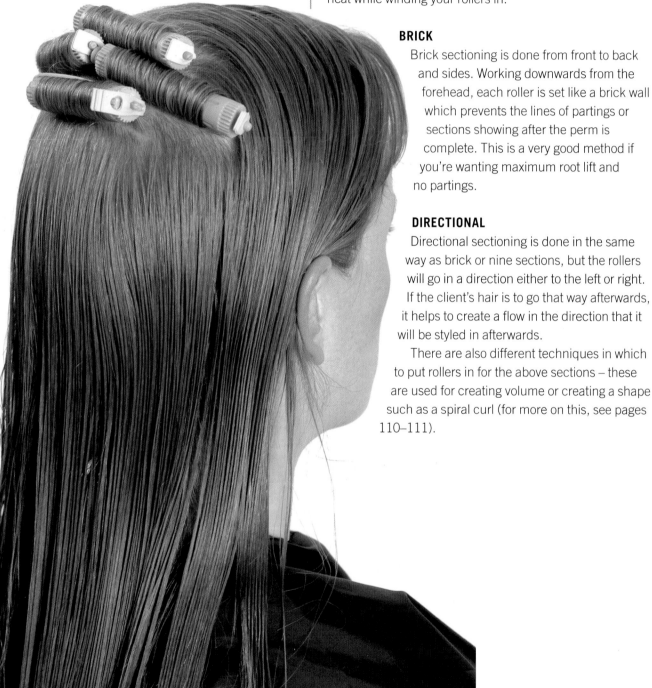

## NINE SECTION

Hair is put into nine sections and each section is taken individually, starting at the neck and working forwards, and divided into sub-sections for each individual roller. Nine section is used as a methodical way to perm most hair, but is mainly used for mid-length to long hair as it helps to keep it neat while winding your rollers in.

## BRICK

Brick sectioning is done from front to back and sides. Working downwards from the forehead, each roller is set like a brick wall which prevents the lines of partings or sections showing after the perm is complete. This is a very good method if you're wanting maximum root lift and no partings.

## DIRECTIONAL

Directional sectioning is done in the same way as brick or nine sections, but the rollers will go in a direction either to the left or right. If the client's hair is to go that way afterwards, it helps to create a flow in the direction that it will be styled in afterwards.

There are also different techniques in which to put rollers in for the above sections – these are used for creating volume or creating a shape such as a spiral curl (for more on this, see pages 110–111).

# Technique

Once all the above is decided, the hair should be shampooed once with a pre-perm shampoo or soft cleansing shampoo to remove oil or excess products. It is then towel dried lightly and prepared into sections to wind into the chosen direction with the rollers selected.

Once wound, the hair should be of even dampness all over. If it is dried out on one side and damp on the other, it will cause a difference with the perm lotion as the water will dilute it if the hair is too wet. Lightly spray the hair with water to make it even. Cotton is used around the client's hairline to stop product from running onto the skin.

In the old days they used to pre-damp hair, which was to apply perm lotion to the hair first, then wind on rollers and allow to develop. In recent years perms have moved on, however, and now we tend to post-damp after the rollers are in. This is also due to the fact that if used correctly, perm lotion (main ingredient ammonium thioglycollate) is only supposed to break down 25 per cent of the disulphide bonds, which is enough to get the right result whilst causing the least damage possible to the hair. If too many bonds are broken, hair becomes weaker – applying lotion before the rollers went on meant that it was on the hair much longer and often broke far too many bonds.

Perm lotion should be applied to every roller and as evenly as possible – make sure you don't miss any. The lotion should be applied from the nape up to the crown – all over the back first, then the sides and finally the top as heat rises from the top of the head and tends to slightly speed up the development. If applied this way, the whole head will be ready at the same time.

Development times vary according to the make of the

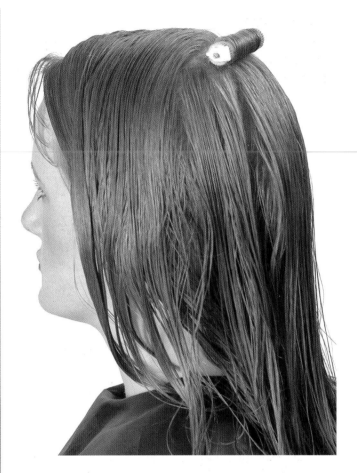

product, so always check manufacturer's instructions before proceeding with any chemical processes. Once the development time is up, neutralizing takes place. This removes the perm lotion from the hair and leaves the bonds temporarily broken. The warmer the client can stand the water, the more easily the lotion is removed, but all the hair must be rinsed thoroughly and evenly for an even result.

Once rinsed, the neutralizer is applied. The neutralizing chemical (main ingredient hydrogen peroxide) rejoins the disulphide bonds to the shape in which you have formed them. Neutralizer normally comes in a liquid or foam consistency, and it must be applied over every roller. All the rollers must be wound to the same tightness for this process, so if some have come loose it is a good time to tighten them. Again, follow the manufacturer's instructions when applying.

Once completed, it is normal procedure to advise a client not to wash or wet the hair for at least 48 hours, as this may relax the perm shape. It takes this amount of time for the hair bonds to settle and also gives the hair time to de-stress, as the chemicals used are quite stressing to the hair and scalp.

## tip

Hair only absorbs a certain amount of liquid, so going over each roller three times (once meaning going over the roller one time, not over and back) is more than enough for hair of any thickness, provided you have not wound too much hair onto the roller. Doing this should also stop too much seepage of the liquid onto the client's skin, which could burn.

# perm and neutralize

Although perming seems to have become almost extinct, it is still important to learn the technique so that, should you be asked to do one, or should they come back into fashion, you are able to oblige.

**APPLY A PERM**

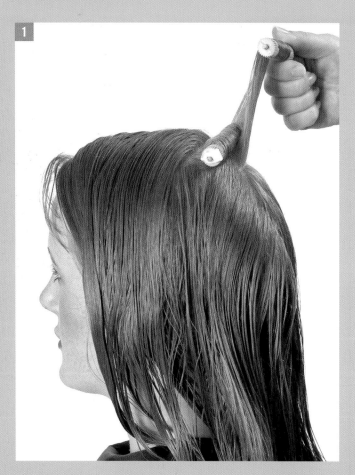

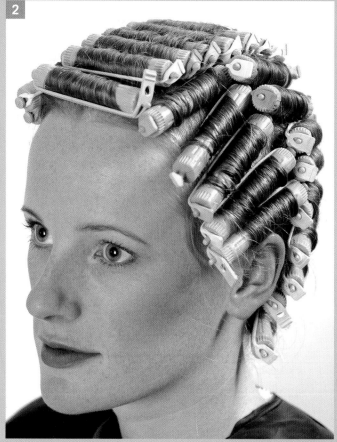

① Pre-wash hair with pre-perm shampoo or a light cleansing shampoo, lightly towel dry and comb through. Put hair into the required sectioning. Take small individual sub-sections and put end papers on the ends of the hair, holding the section taut. Put the roller onto the end paper and wind down slowly, keeping the hair taut.

② Continue doing the same to all the hair. Once complete, lightly damp a length – enough to wrap around the head – of cotton wool. Secure around the outside edge of the rollers around the head, taking it behind the ears and secure in a knot at the nape.

Apply the lotion after selecting the lotion type in consultation with the client. The lotion will spray out in a line from the end of the bottle – spray each roller three times starting at the nape and doing the front last. If not all the lotion is used, do not use it just for the sake of it as it will go on to the scalp and possibly burn it.

③ Once dampened with perm lotion, develop for the time recommended by the manufacturer. Once developed, remove the cotton wool and take the client to the back wash. Protecting the face from the water running down it, rinse the rollers for a good 5 minutes (or according to the manufacturer's instructions), making sure to rinse all the rollers well.

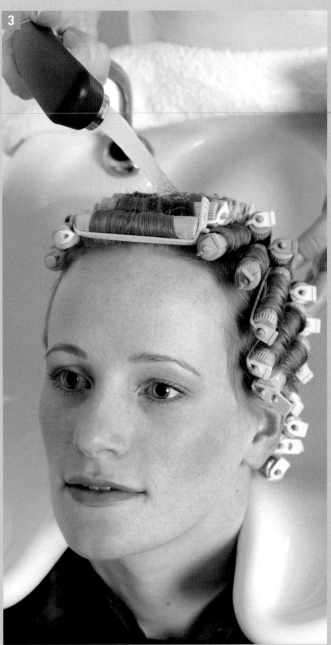

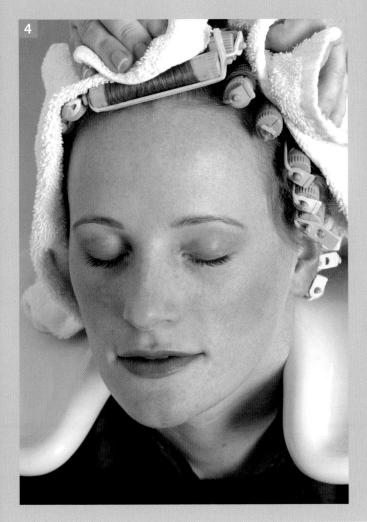

④ Once rinsed, lightly towel dry by pressing down on the rollers with a towel to remove excess water.

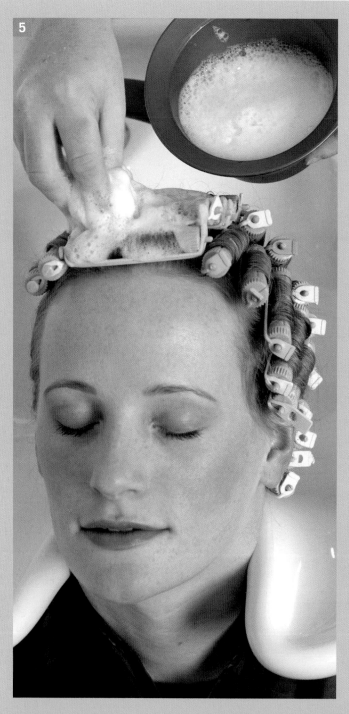

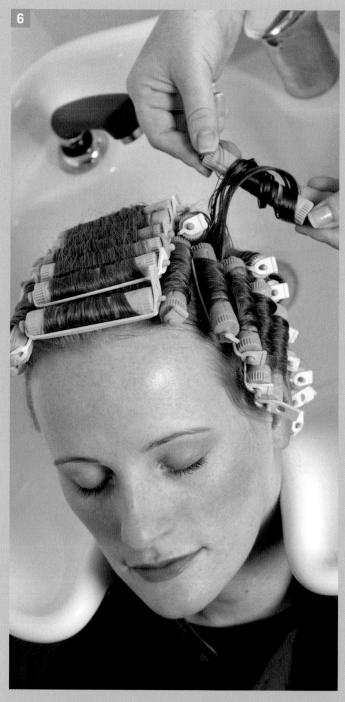

⑤ Apply the neutralizer according to the individual manufacturer's instructions and allow it to develop for around 5–7 minutes.

⑥ Remove the rollers without pulling or tugging, so as to cause as little strain on the hair as possible. Lightly rinse the hair with water only (do NOT use shampoo), then towel dry and style as required.

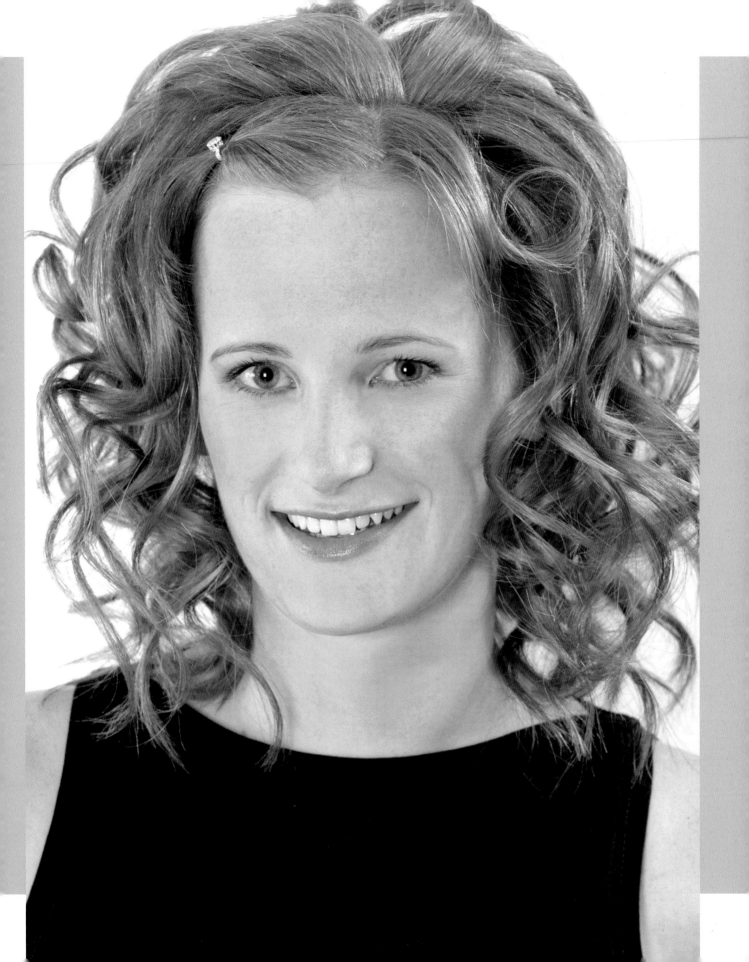

# different winds

There are many different sectioning techniques and winds that you can use when perming, depending on the result you wish to achieve. Listed here are a few of the more popular ones.

## Brick

Start at the front and wind two rollers straight back in the normal nine section manner. Then continue winding back in a brick-laying manner all the way through the sides, top and back. This wind helps to reduce tram lines in the final style.

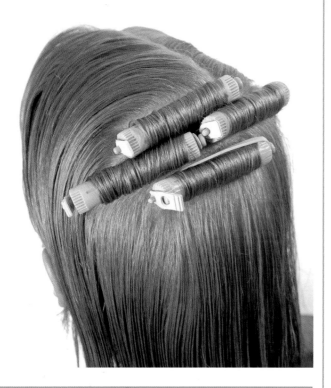

## Nine section

Using a selected perm roller, start winding preferably at the front or at the nape section in the chosen wind. Work through each section until all nine sections (see page 85 for pattern) are complete and in line. This is the method shown in the step-by-step instructions on the previous pages.

## Directional

Winding either in brick formation or general nine section pattern, wind the rollers to a side or in the direction in which hair may go, not always as going back. This will direct the flow of hair and make it easier to style in that direction.

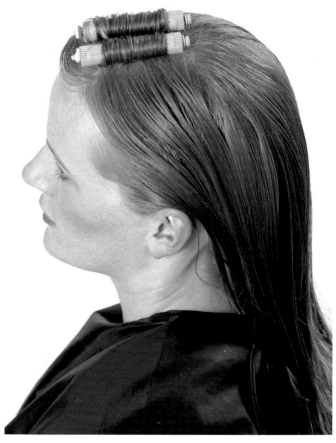

## tip

### FOR BRICK SECTIONING

You must have the ends of the hair wound right around the roller and not bending backwards the other way – this will create a permanent fish hook effect and can only be removed by cutting.

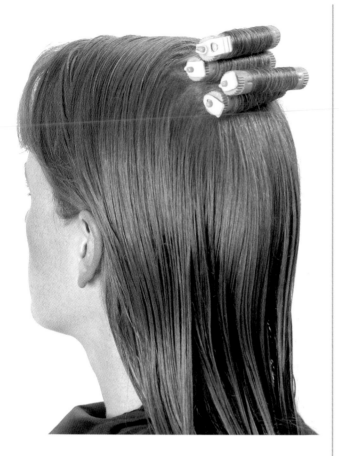

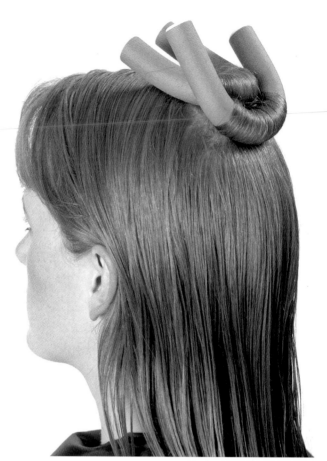

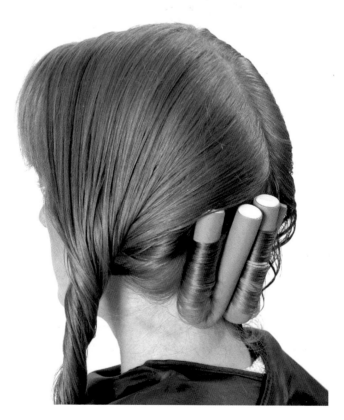

## Piggy back

This technique is a little more intricate. Take a regular perm section and split it into two. Put the back half in one roller and the front in another, but pull the front one over the top of the back one, This creates great root lift and works well if two roller sizes are used, the slightly larger one on the underneath and a smaller one on top.

## Molton Brown regular wind

This can be used with a nine section, brick or directional sectioning. Using the softer, bendy Molton Brown roller gives a softer curl and and does not leave tram lines in the hair.

## Molton Brown spiral wind

This is used on vertical sections, starting at the nape and working up to create a spiral or corkscrew wind. The effect shows a little, but all perms need work when styling – don't be misled into thinking that you can wash it and leave it for this spiral curl to be perfect.

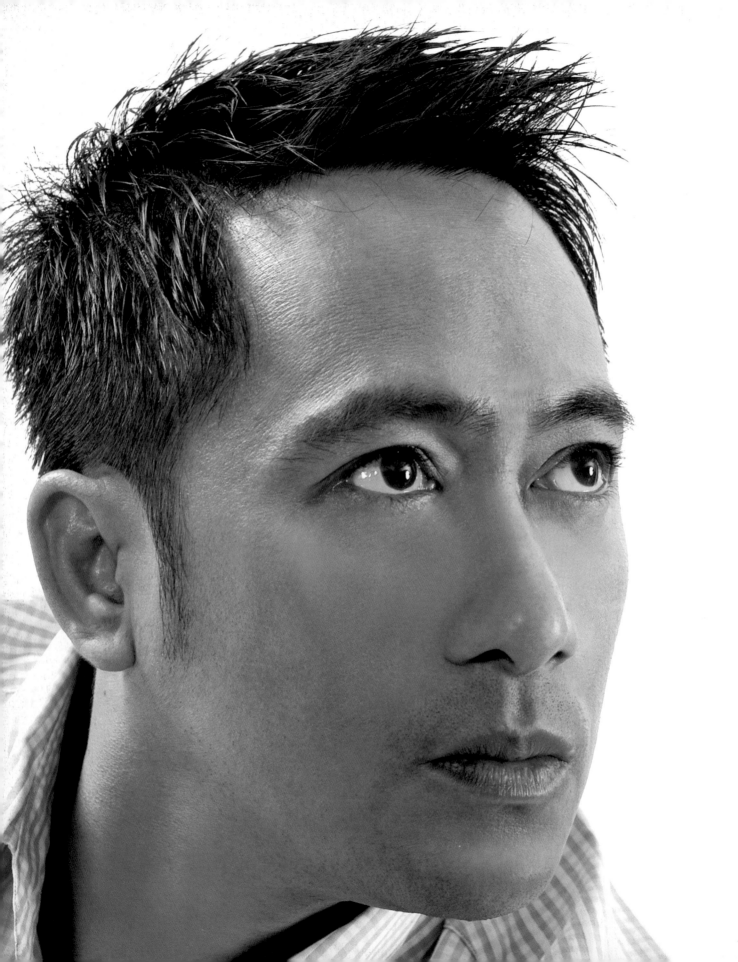

# 04 the male

# cutting men's hair

In the past, men's hairdressing was very different, using old barbering techniques including cut-throat razor shaves, hot face towels and a short back and sides carried out with clippers. However, as with all hairdressing, this has changed dramatically and men's haircuts are now very versatile – even feminine in some ways, as men's hair can be almost any length and requires many of the same cutting techniques as women's hair.

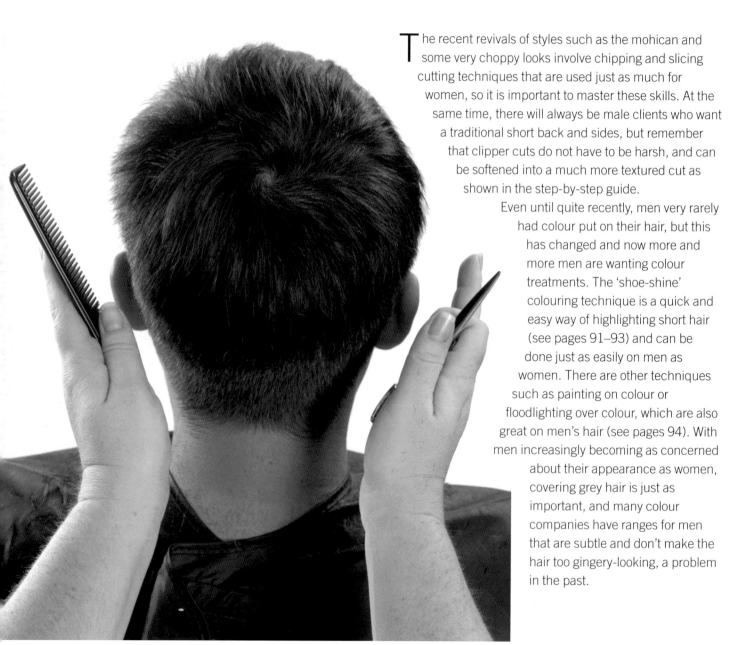

The recent revivals of styles such as the mohican and some very choppy looks involve chipping and slicing cutting techniques that are used just as much for women, so it is important to master these skills. At the same time, there will always be male clients who want a traditional short back and sides, but remember that clipper cuts do not have to be harsh, and can be softened into a much more textured cut as shown in the step-by-step guide.

Even until quite recently, men very rarely had colour put on their hair, but this has changed and now more and more men are wanting colour treatments. The 'shoe-shine' colouring technique is a quick and easy way of highlighting short hair (see pages 91–93) and can be done just as easily on men as women. There are other techniques such as painting on colour or floodlighting over colour, which are also great on men's hair (see pages 94). With men increasingly becoming as concerned about their appearance as women, covering grey hair is just as important, and many colour companies have ranges for men that are subtle and don't make the hair too gingery-looking, a problem in the past.

# men's cut

Clippers for men's hair generally come with plastic graded guides (usually numbered one to four) that are added to the end of the clippers and determine how short the hair is cut. A grade four cut would leave the hair a little longer, while a grade one would be very short – almost 1 mm. Always determine with the client what grade they would like before beginning.

## how to...

### CUT MEN'S HAIR

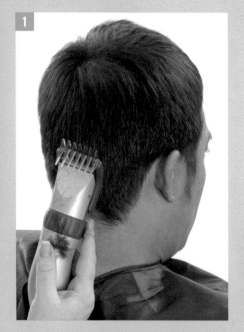

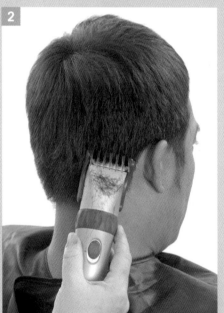

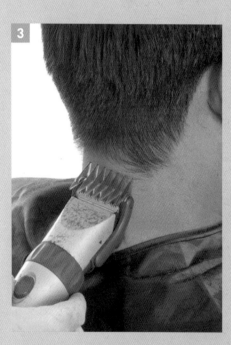

① Having established the overall length desired, start at the back of neck with a large grade and work up the head to the occipital bone, which graduates out of the head as you get closer to the crown. Doing this will allow you to gradually take a shorter graduation as you work down closer to the hair line, without creating a line in the hair.

② Slowly take the clippers up the hair and bring them out at the desired point of blending (where the longer hair on top meets the shorter hair at the back and sides). Do this around the head on the back and sides, remembering when doing the sides to take the clippers up to the same point as before on the back, and not further up.

③ Once you have done this, repeat using the next grade up. Do not go all the way up to where you were before – this will make the graduation down into the neck and sides near the ear more gradual.

▷

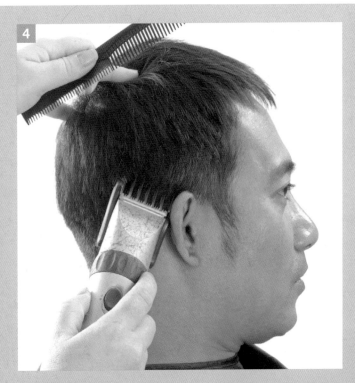

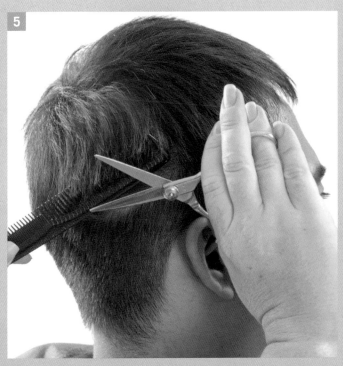

④ Repeat again on the next grade up to make it even closer cut into the next line area, but again only take up just a little. If done correctly you will end up with a soft, graduated hair cut into the neck and sides.

⑤ Now you have to blend the area that you stopped at by using a scissor over comb technique and gently removing any bulk or length.

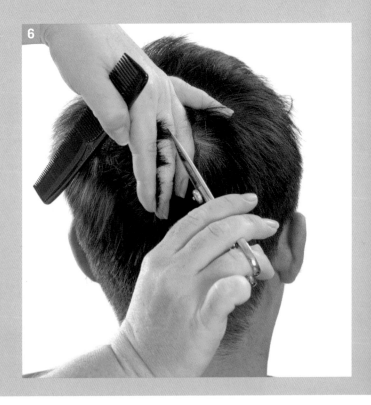

⑥ You can also chip cut scissor over comb, but do it very lightly or you will create large marks of weight in short hair.

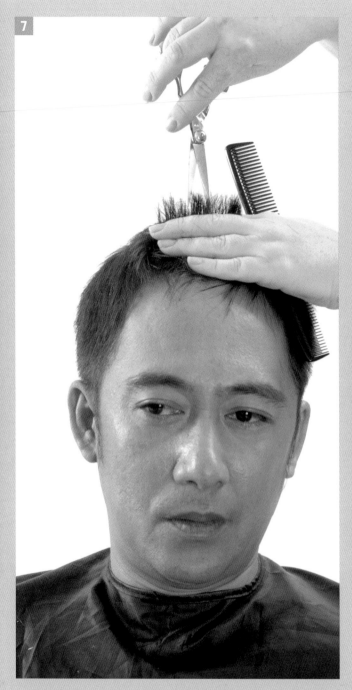

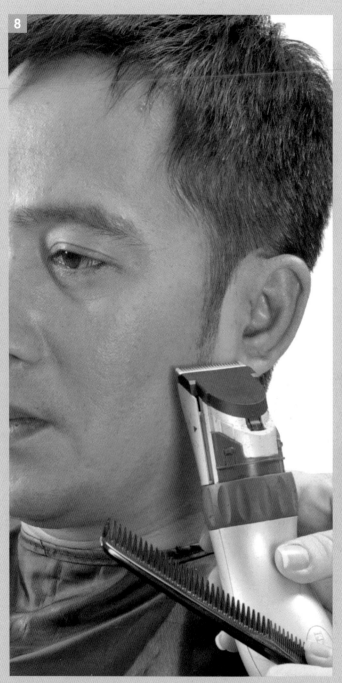

⑦ The top is then blended by taking small sections and chip cutting the top area to create a choppy look.

⑧ Now you need to clean the hairline and around the ears. Start at the front on the sideburns and cut straight to the desired length. It is best to cut the other side straight away, but measure carefully and make sure that they are the same length.

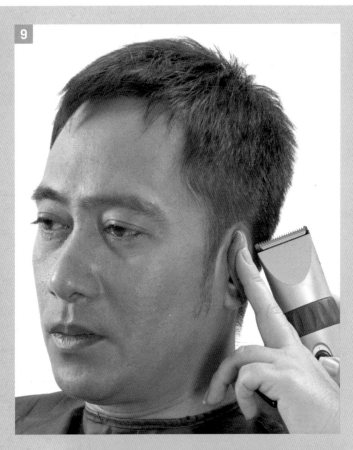

⑨ Now work with a steady hand to remove excess hair from the sideburn up to the top of the ear. Pull the ear forward and do the same behind the ear right the way down to the nape area. Do the same to the other side.

## tip

Do not cut into the growth line of the hair as this spoils the cut. Just remove hair that is longer. Some men may have extreme hair growth on the neck so it is impossible not to cut into the hair growth line, but do so gradually with clippers first when starting this cut.

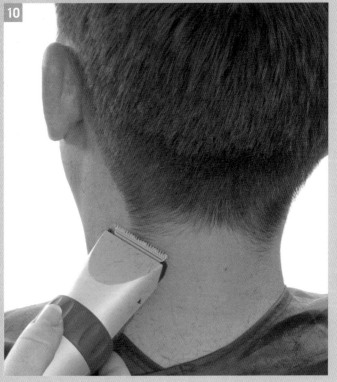

⑩ Facing the client forward, assess the neck hair growth and lightly remove to create a neat neck line. There are three ways to cut a man's neck line: square, round or tapered. Square and rounded are fairly self-explanatory, whilst tapered is gradual, with no visible line of hair as to where it stops and starts. Once you have finished, style as required.

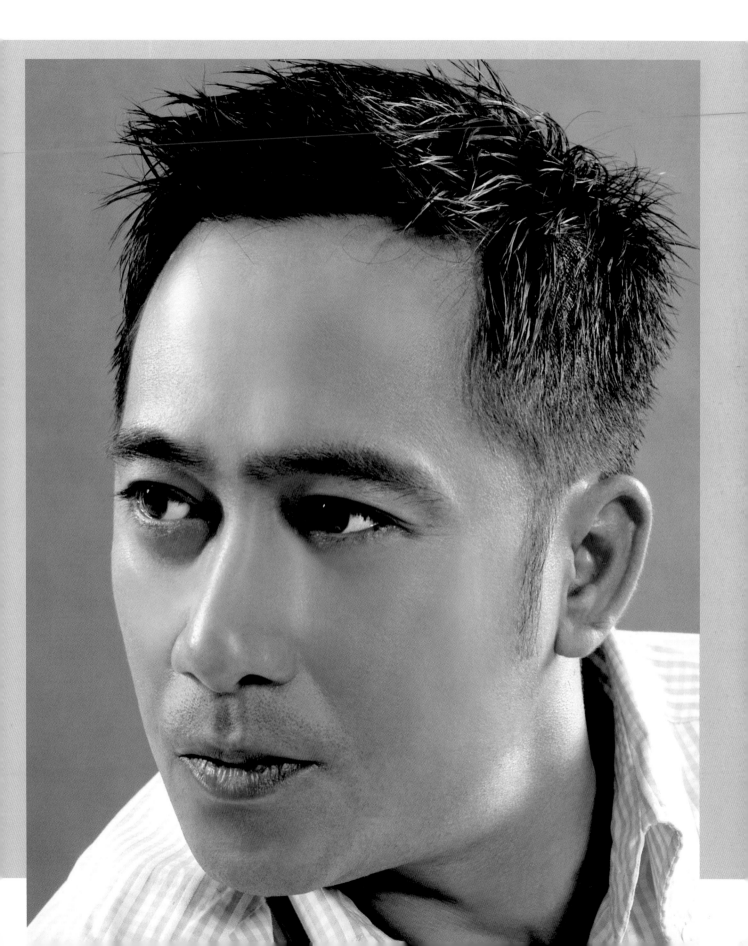

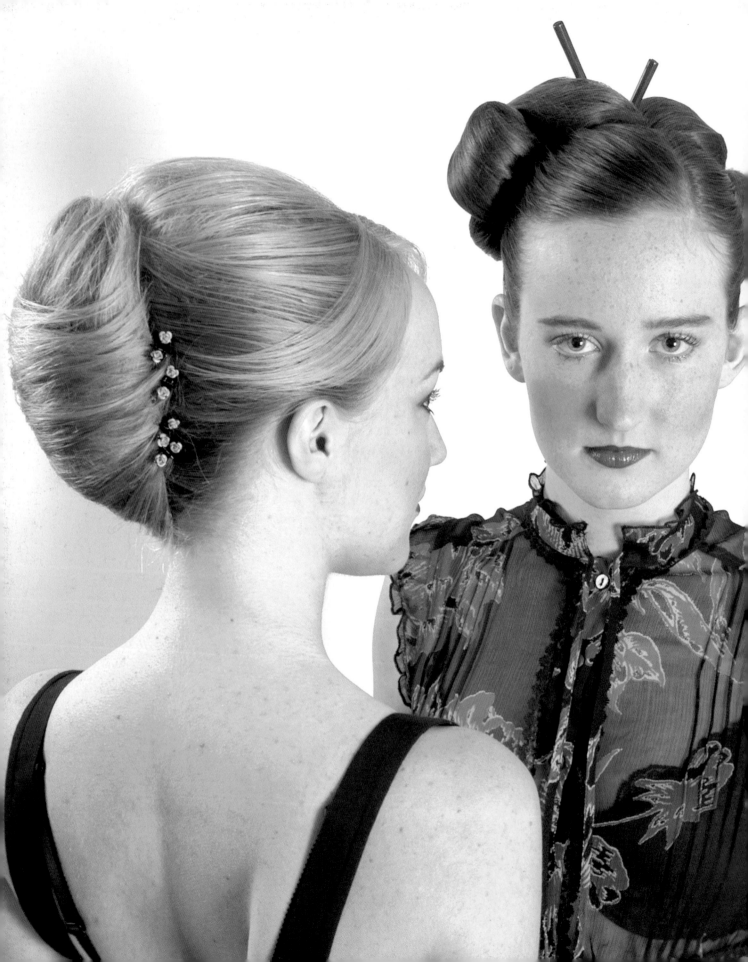

# 05 formal invite

# formal hair

When dressing long hair for formal occasions, your first step is, of course, to find out what the occasion in question is – whether it's a wedding, cocktail party, special dinner or a fancy dress or period party. The occasion should immediately conjure up ideas of what style of hair might be appropriate. In this section we will introduce you to a few essential tools to have handy for dressing long hair into formal hairstyles, and take you through three different formal ideas.

There are some essential things to remember when dressing formal hair.

★ Always practice your style prior to the day of the event. This will help you to get an idea of how long the style takes, how easy or otherwise it is, and help to ensure that you are creating the right look for the client's needs.

★ Make sure that on the day of the hairstyling the client wears appropriate clothing that does not need to be pulled off over the masterpiece you have just created!

★ Find out what type of outfit the client will be wearing. It is not always a good idea to have the hair dressed down if there is going to be a lot of detail around the neck, as it will cover it. Alternatively, dresses with no straps can be very revealing of the neck, so they may require some pieces of hair to be left down. Either of these scenarios could affect the style you have in mind.

★ Hair accessories – are there any that the client wishes to use? This is crucial to find out as it can alter the look completely, so the formal hair should be designed around them.

★ Remember to remind the client that sometimes formal hair can look strange with no makeup and without the dress they will be wearing, so bear this in mind when practicing and reassure them that it will look stunning when done for the occasion.

★ Never over-use products on formally dressed hair even if you are putting all of it up, as if you need to re-do a part of it during the process, it is very hard to move hair that is stuck up with hairspray or product.

★ Backcombing is a vital for most long hair formal styles and is a useful technique to learn and practice. It can help tremendously when dressing formal hair, giving body and hold without using too many products. Try not to do it too often, though – over time it can damage the cuticle.

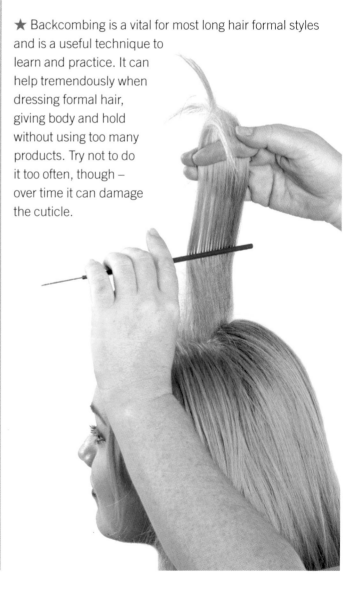

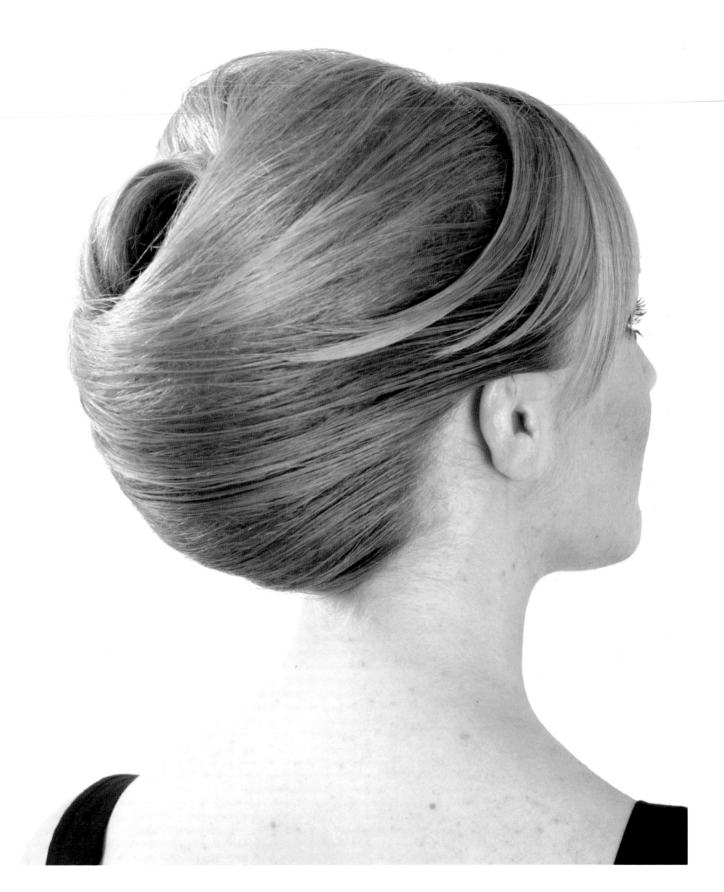

# equipment

There are some items that will make doing formal hair much easier. Make sure you have everything that you will need to hand before beginning. Set up a trolley and make sure that all your tools are within easy reach.

## Pins

### KIRBY PINS

These pins are the main holding grip for most hair-ups. They are strong and can be the backbone of a formal hairstyle. You can buy cheaper makes of kirby pin that don't tend to be so strong, so avoid these and buy the best. The prongs of the pin should stay together and not separate once in place – on cheaper makes, once the prongs are spread apart to be put into the hair, they do not close, and therefore do not hold the hair well.

### PRONG PINS

These grips are used for pinning the hair into the finished shape, as they can be hidden well, unlike kirby pins. They come in different thicknesses and the very thin ones are excellent for hiding and holding the ends of the hair.

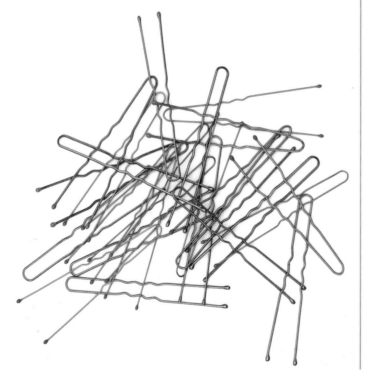

| tip | |
| --- | --- |

Don't use regular elastic bands as they break and snap the hair. They are made for paper and other tough materials, not hair, so to avoid damage, never use them.

## Hair bands

These come in many forms and many materials. The most popular sort to use at the moment look like elastic but are a soft rubber and come in many shades. The best shade to use, of course, is either a colour the same as the hair colour, or translucent so that they cannot be seen. You don't want people to see any of the infrastructure beneath your beautiful creation – it should look effortless.

## Hair nets

The best type of nets to use for formal hairstyles are very thin, fine nets that are made of fine denier like tights and stockings. You can hardly see them in the hair, but they are invaluable when putting up long hair.

## Accessories

Accessories come in so many shapes and sizes, from clips, hair bands and tiaras to flowers, ribbons, crystals and even pearls and diamonds. Accessories are a great way to dress up beautiful formal hair, but don't overdo it. Adding too much can result in the client looking like a Christmas tree. Remember that formal is elegant!

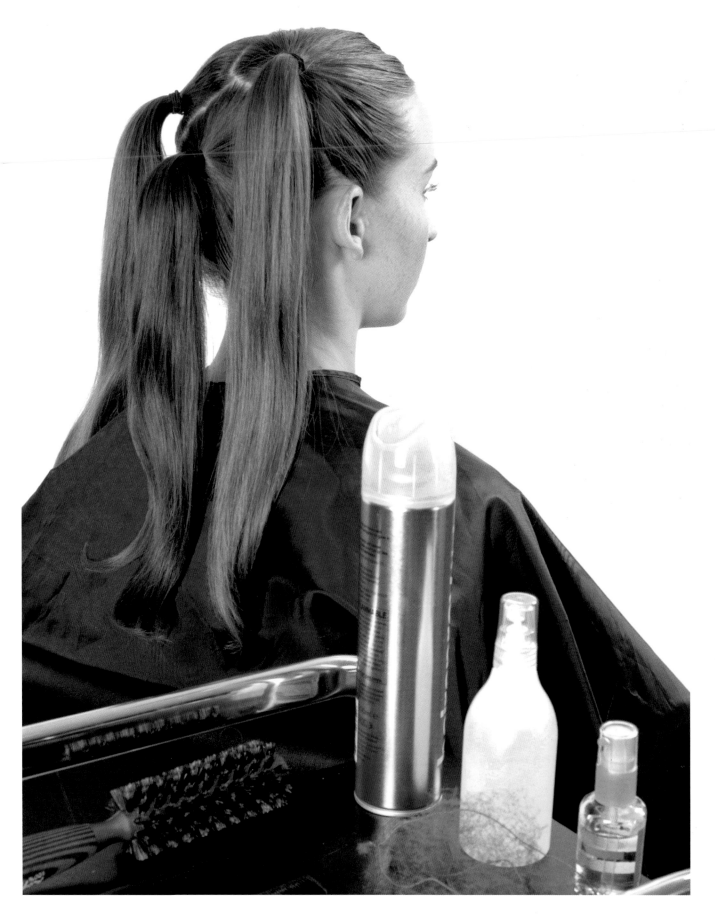

# look 1: the low roll

This hairstyle is very versatile and can be as sophisticated or as dressed-up as you wish. By adding accessories, it can be used both for bridal parties or more simple occasions.

## how to...

**CREATE A LOW ROLL**

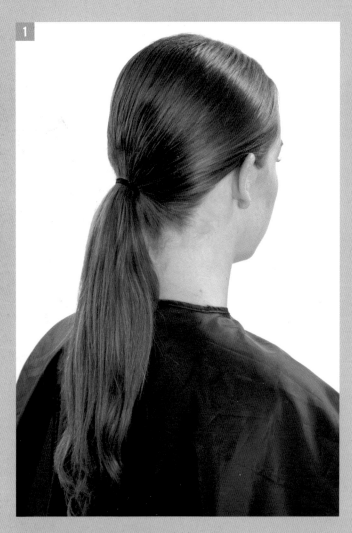

① Hair should either have been washed the previous day or already set on heated rollers. Smooth the hair down to the nape and put firmly into an elastic.

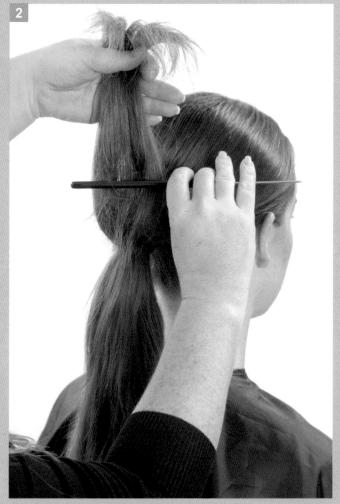

② Taking the hair into separate sub-sections, backcomb gently from root to tip.

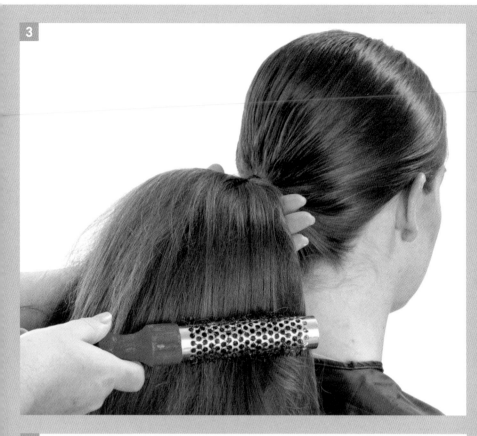

③ Once backcombed, smooth over the top of the hair ensuring that there are no lumps. Spray with a little light hairspray.

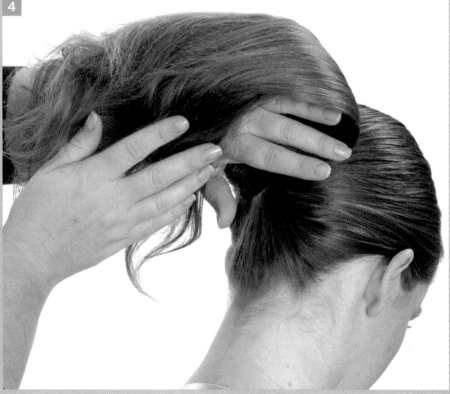

④ Push the client's head as far forward as possible and flip the hair over towards the forehead.

⑤ **Pin the hair against the head in a semi-circlular shape. Once the pins are secure, bring the client's head back to the normal position.**

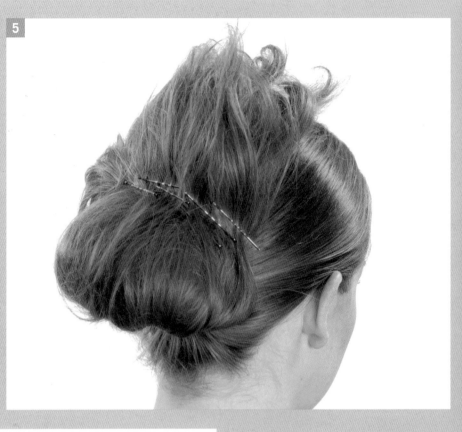

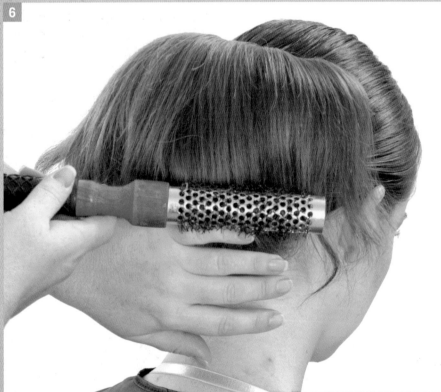

⑥ **Smooth the hair with a soft brush and tuck it round and under into a roll in the middle.**

⑦ **Pin the hair into place with prong pins wherever needed.**

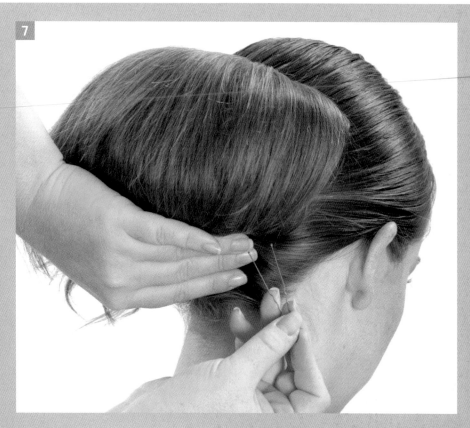

⑧ **Smooth the hair and tuck the ends under on each side, blending with the middle section and pinning with prong pins all round to secure.**

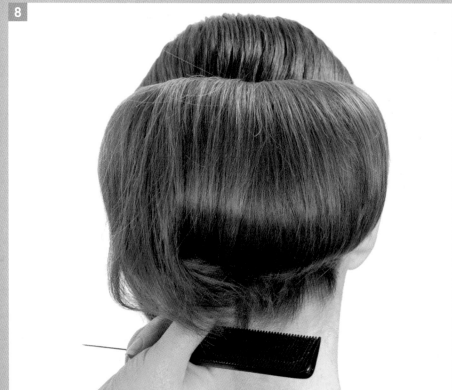

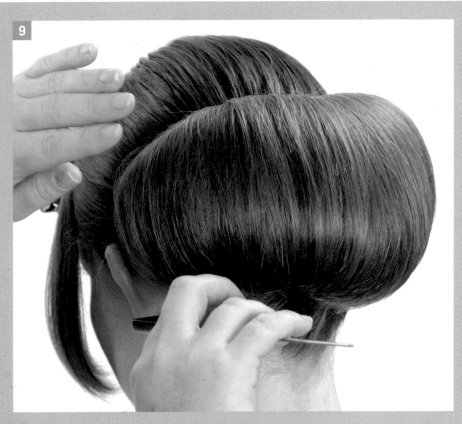

⑨ Lightly spray with hairspray and make sure all the hair is secure, smoothing and finishing where needed.

⑩ Backcomb and style the fringe area, if needed, securing with hairspray once smoothed and in place.

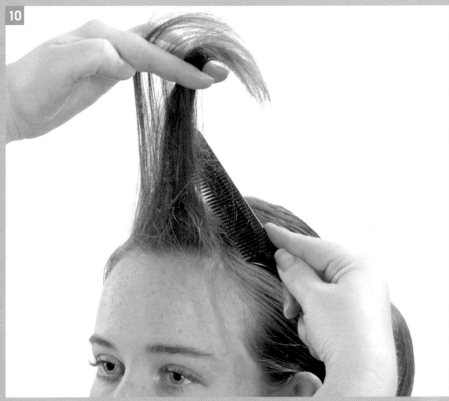

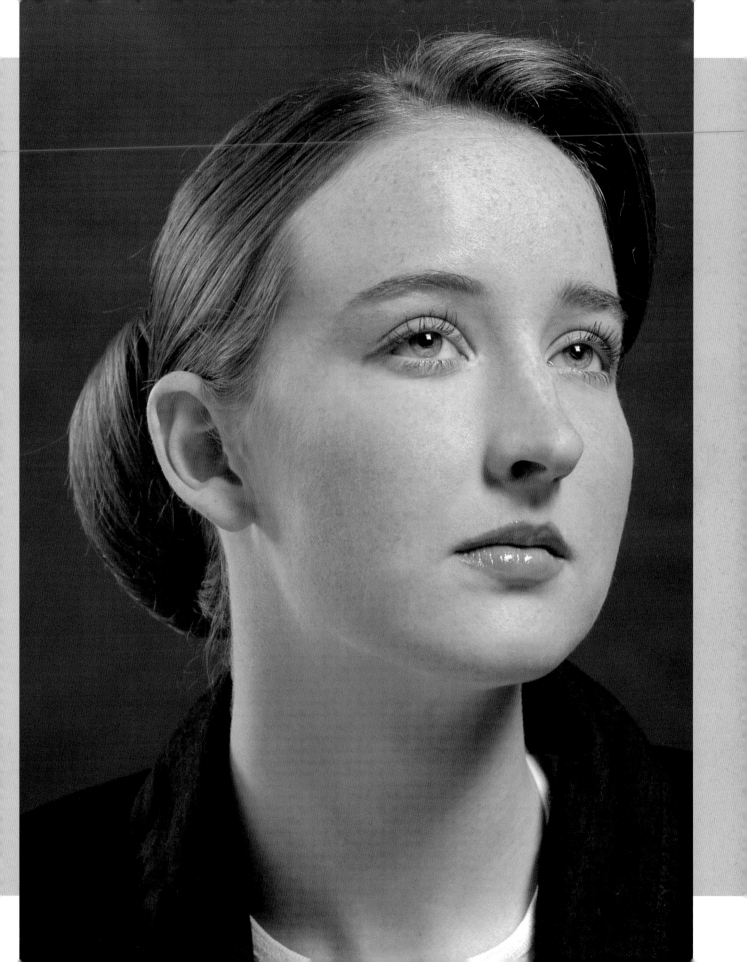

# look 2: the pleat

The classic pleat has been around for many years, but it is a style that needs lots of practice to execute perfectly. This is another versatile look, perfect for parties, a night on the town or a bride-to-be.

## how to...

**CREATE A PLEAT**

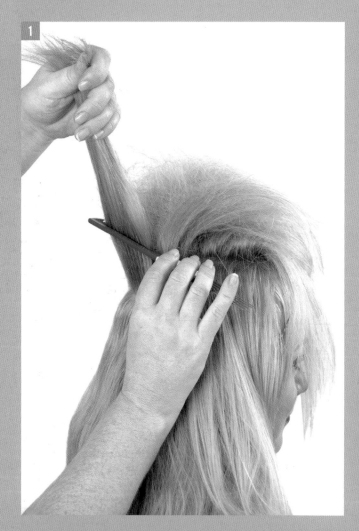

① Hair should have been washed the previous day and be brushed through thoroughly. Taking individual sections from the front to the nape, backcomb the hair from roots to ends.

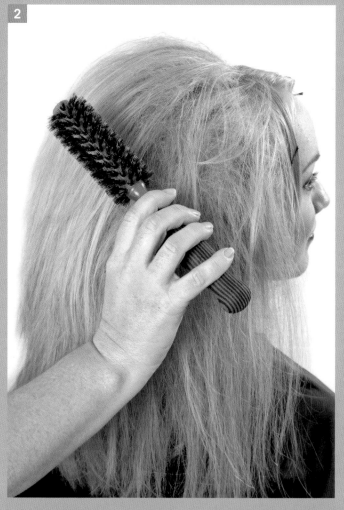

② Once all the hair is backcombed, spray lightly with fine hairspray and, using a soft brush, lightly comb the top of the hair so that it is smooth.

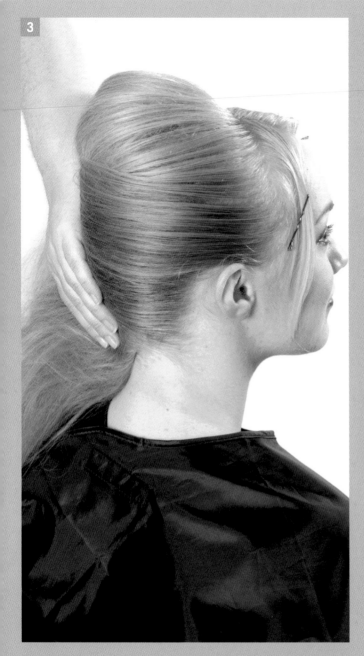

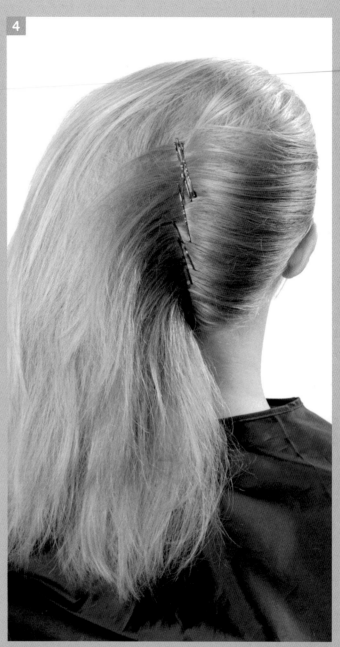

③ Smoothing the right side (or whichever is more comfortable to you), use your other hand to hold the hair into place – this side is to be pinned first.

④ Pin with kirby grips slightly off centre, to your left (or to your right if you started with the left side). Pin right up to near the crown area.

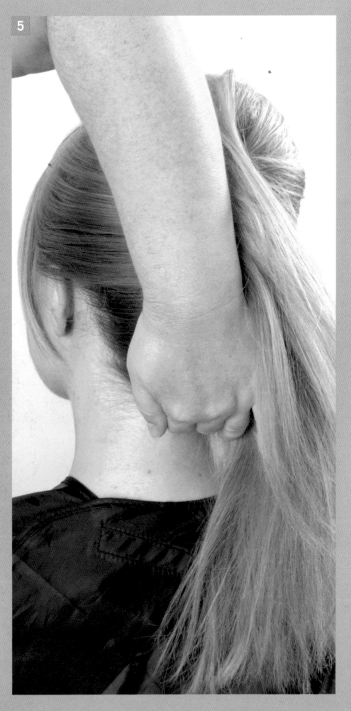

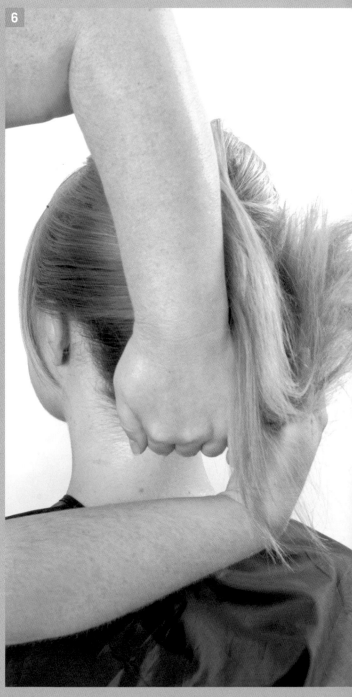

⑤ Taking the other side that is left out and smoothing the top all the time, start to bring it around to the centre again using the back of your arm to hold it in place.

⑥ Once it is in the centre, flip the ends of the hair under to make the pleat roll.

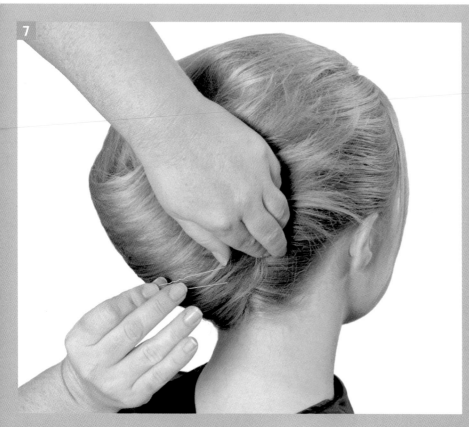

⑦ Using a prong pin (a thicker one), lightly slide the pin in facing outwards first and then sliding it back under the hair. Do this all the way up to secure the whole roll.

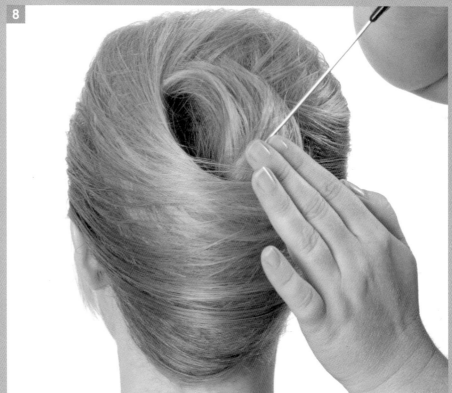

⑧ Once secure, smooth and clean up the whole roll with a soft brush and fine prong pins. Using a tail comb, gently manipulate the top hair inside the roll.

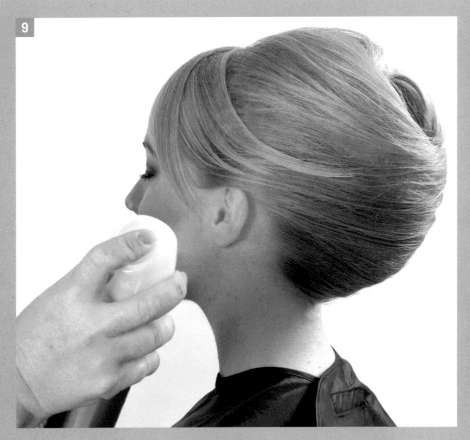

**9** Manipulate and smooth your finished look and tuck in any stray ends, using hairspray where necessary. Use the end of a tail comb to pick out areas that are slightly flat.

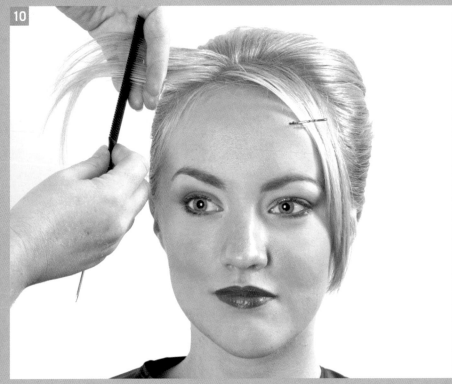

**10** Style the fringe and front areas, if necessary, backcombing for added volume and then smoothing down and fixing with hairspray.

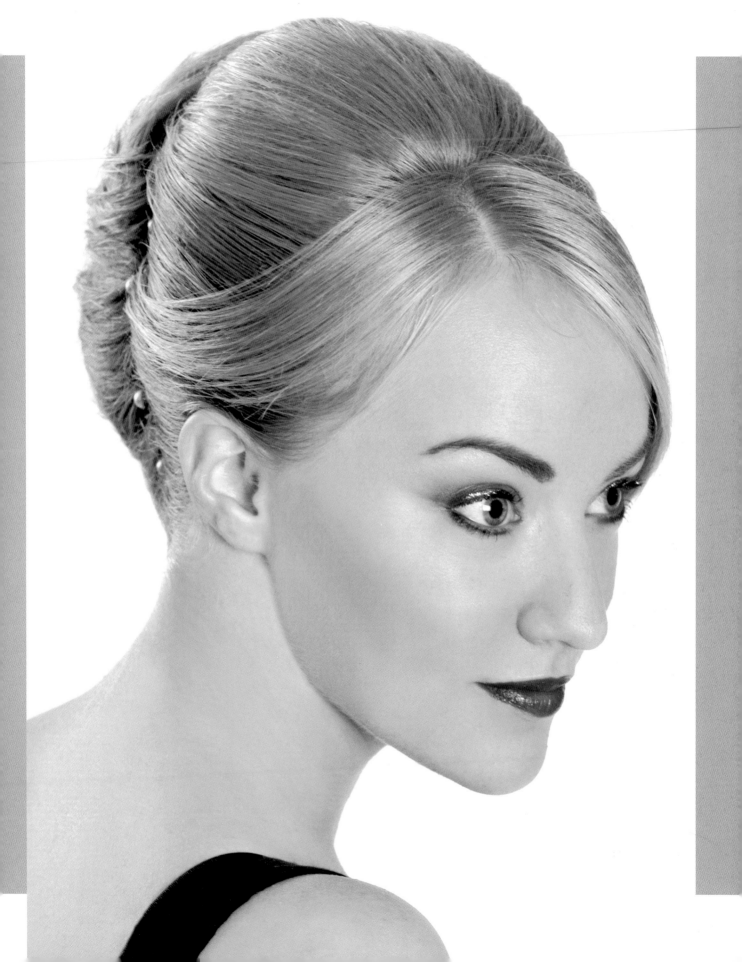

# look 3: the twist

Twists are not a commonly used formal hairstyle and for this reason can look very striking and unusual. They will be slightly different every time you do them, and again they are suitable for many different occasions.

## how to...

### CREATE A TWIST

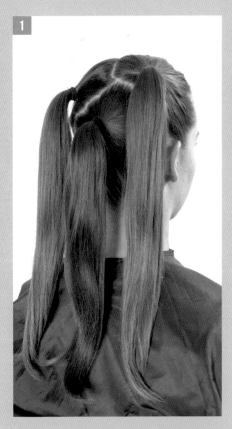

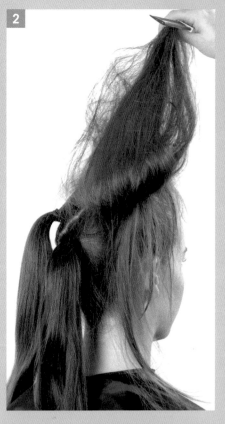

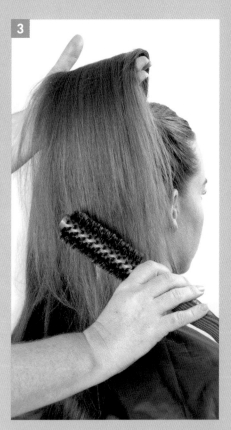

① Hair should have been washed the previous day. Divide the hair neatly into three even ponytails. It is your choice as to where they are located, depending on where you want the finished hair to sit. Once the ponytails are secure, lightly spray to fix any loose hairs.

② Take one of the ponytails at the front and, in small sections, backcomb the whole of the ponytail. Spray the backcombing lightly once done.

③ Gently smooth out the surface of the backcombed ponytail with a soft brush and lightly spray once done.

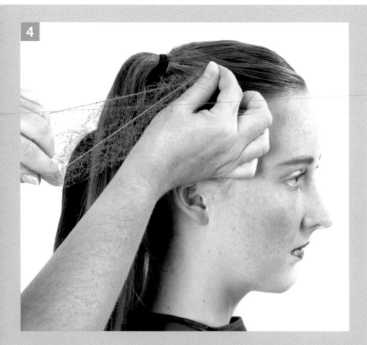

④ Put a kirby grip through a fine coloured hairnet (preferably the same colour as the client's hair) and attach it securely to the top of the ponytail.

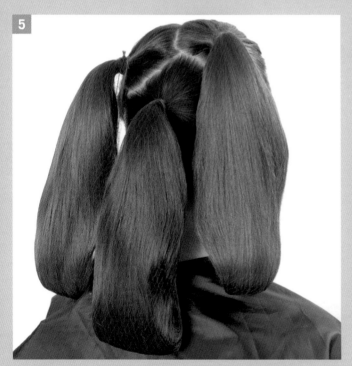

⑤ Put the ponytail securely into the net and lightly push it forward, out of the way. Follow this same procedure with all three ponytails.

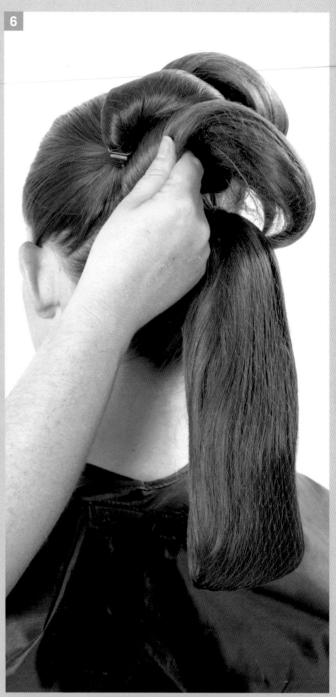

⑥ Start with the ponytail closest to the front, manipulating it into twists and curls. This will happen differently every time you do this style, as it is imposible to create the exact same waves every time. The effect you get depends on the hair's movement that day, but the results will always be similar.

▷

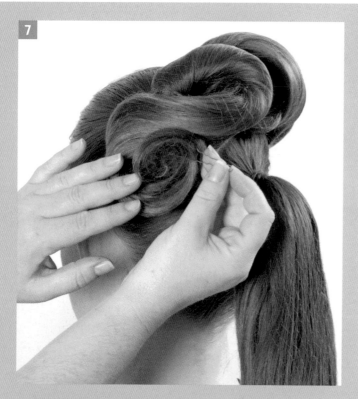

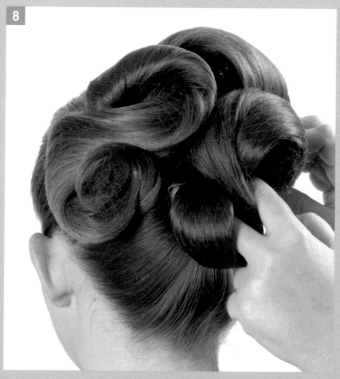

⑦ Create the shape you want by manipulating it with your hands before pinning securely. Ensure that the pins and elastics are well hidden. Do the same with the other two ponytails.

⑧ Stand back now and again to get a better view as you arrange the hair. Try not to pin any hair close to the hairline, as it makes it harder to cover the elastic near the roots.

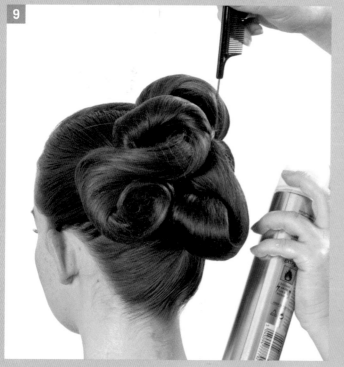

## tip

If you want the hair to look like a hat, bring all the ponytails to a side. It also looks good with all the ponytails at the back and kept low on the head. This look can be done with as many ponytails as you want – just make sure they are of the same thickness or it can look uneven.

⑨ Smooth down any frizzy hairs with a little hairspray and use a tail comb to tuck the curls into place. This style looks good both on its own or dressed with hair accessories – just don't get too carried away!

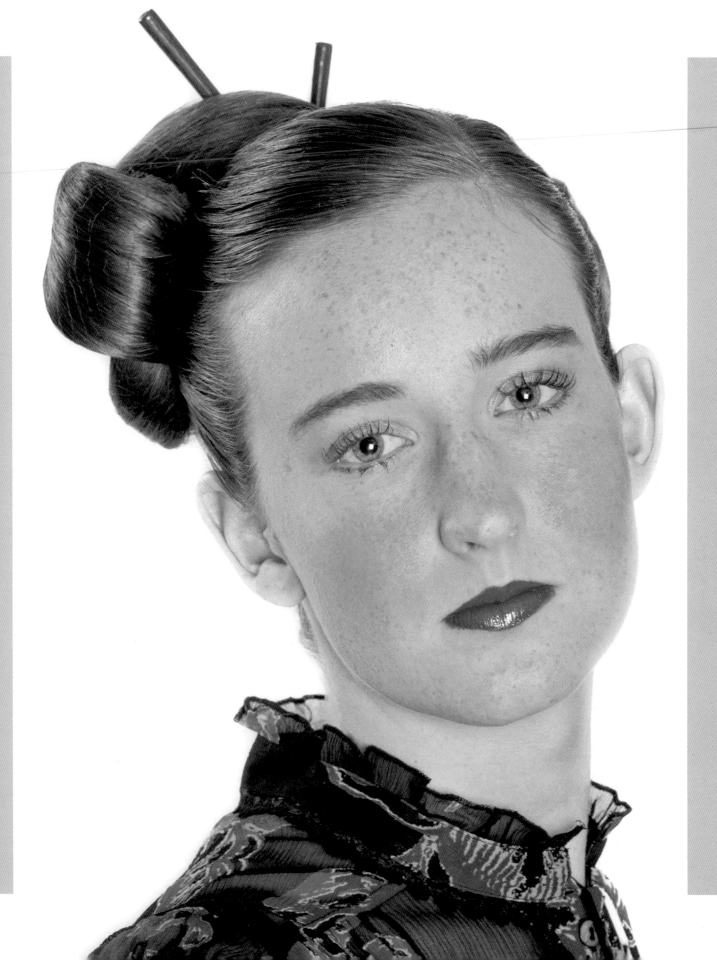

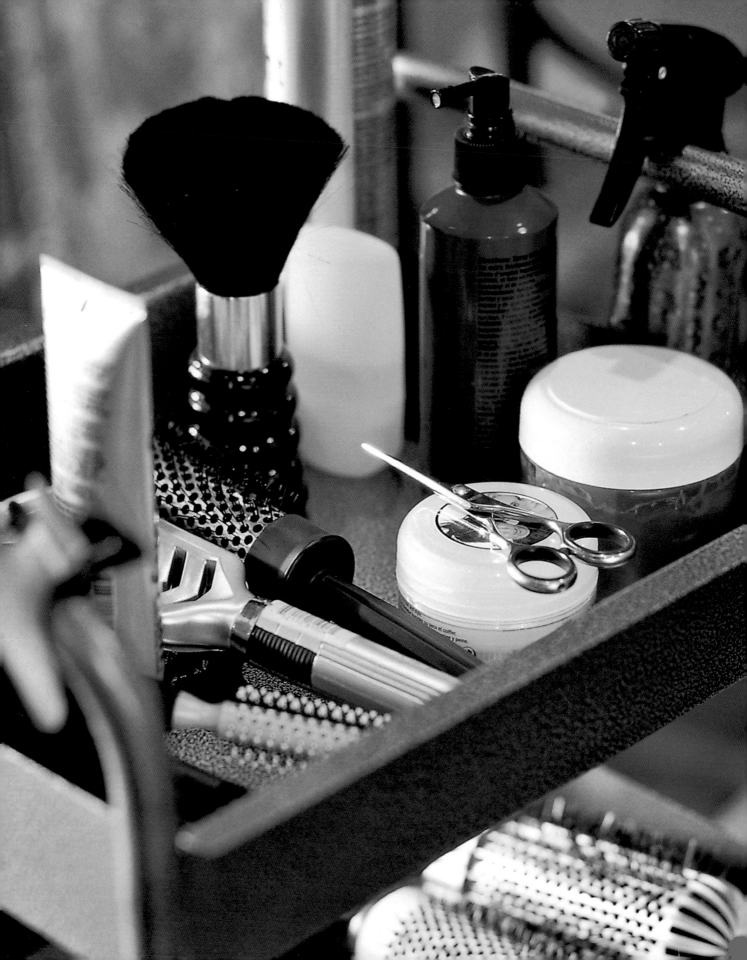

# 06 salon genius

# business potential

As a salon owner, there are ways of making everybody in the team highly skilled money-makers, and with good working practice your business could have great potential. Motivating your staff can be hard work, but very rewarding.

## Retaining loyalty

Clients come into your salon for a reason: often they have been before and are returning or regular clients; some are casual walk-in or new clients; others are 'floaters' and come in now and again but to different stylists. All of these are potential money-makers and must be dealt with, with care.

The problem with most salons is that they become complacent with regular clients. They often dazzle new clients to encourage them then into becoming regular customers, but once they are regular they become complacent with them too. If a client is known by name, sat down and asked if they want 'the usual', they will often say yes, not knowing how to ask for a change. The client will eventually become bored and go somewhere else, where a new and exciting hairstyle might be more forthcoming. Many

salons lose a large number of clients because of this, and it's something you need to address if you are to be successful. The trick is to treat all clients the same as the first day they came in. Don't be complacent and imagine that you will always have that client and their custom.

Clients can be extremely loyal if they get a great service every time they come in, so inspire them by always suggesting new ideas. Even if they don't accept, you have offered them a chance to go for something different, which will keep them coming back. You can even treat a regular client to occasional freebies (within reason) – although always check with the manager first. A simple free treatment or extra-long head massage can make a huge difference from a client's perspective. Be careful not to overdo this though, and do make sure to mention that it is a special treat

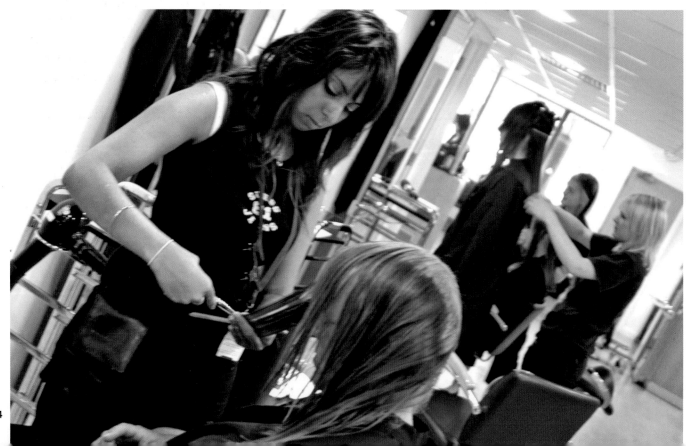

for being a loyal customer – you will find that there are always some clients who try to take advantage and get the same treatment every time without paying extra.

Promotions or loyalty offers are also a great way of getting customers to stay with you – much like some coffee shops, you can stamp a card for every haircut they have with you and they get the tenth one free, or half price.

Above all, be sure to make a fuss of all your clients – after all, they are the ones who pay your wages.

## Up-selling

A good way of making extra money is to up-sell. For instance, when a client comes in to have a treatment or service done, up-sell that service by one, or even two or three levels. This can be done in several ways:

★Recommend them a product
★ Make the cut into a re-style
★ Change the blow-dry into a cut and blow-dry
★ Suggest a colour treatment
★ Flash a few floodlights on to a men's haircut

Or of course, get them to book their next appointment, which will ensure they come back and spend more money in your salon. Always be sure, however, that the client is fully aware of the costs involved and that they are happy for you to proceed.

All these ideas will increase a client's potential spend. If it works on every client that comes in the door, this can make a big difference to the day's takings or to the targets that each stylist has been set for the day, but don't be too pushy and don't do this every time.

## Target setting

If you have staff, it is a good idea to give them incentives or even yourself if you get paid in commission, which many hairdressers do. Give yourself targets depending on how much you need to make to get the profits to a certain place, or to take home a certain amount of commission. Breaking up targets into weeks or days is even better and will be easier for your staff to grasp.

Targets are a good way of pushing people to their limits, and all levels of staff can take part. You can even split your staff into groups (for instance a stylist and an assistant) and set team incentives to make it more fun and encourage good team-work.

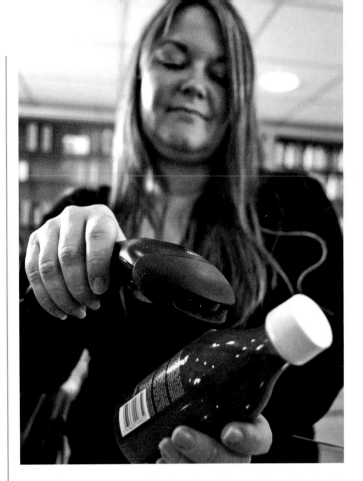

## Retailing

Training your staff regarding the products you use and sell can be a huge advantage, as they will do a much better selling job if they know what each one does and who it would be useful for. We are not all natural sales people, though, and retailing (prescribing and recommending products) is not the easiest of things to do.

It may help if you view it a different way: if your car breaks down, you go to a garage to fix it and they may also tell you what to use to prevent the problem happening again. In the same way, people come to you – the professional – to fix their hair and to advise them on what is best for it in the future.

You can also view from a personal standpoint: you would not want to spend a lot of time and money having a colour done that will fade if you are not recommended the correct product to make it last as long as possible. If you decide not to purchase it then that is your own choice, but you can't say that you weren't warned.

So see it as advice rather than cold-blooded mercenary tactics! Eliminate your client's problems by offering advice on certain products that would benefit them, and avoid the hard sell, which will only alienate the client.

# appearance and customer care

Clients are always attracted to clean environments with polite, courteous and well-mannered staff with good service standards. Good customer service should be your highest priority, so make sure that all your staff are aware of how important this is. In a salon this can start from the moment a client walks in the door or even before.

Nobody likes to walk into a building or room with which they are not familiar – it makes them feel uncomfortable and can be very daunting. Making the entrance of any business that serves the public enticing is crucial. It should be set out to welcome and should never have too many people congregating in the entrance area – this is very off-putting and can deter someone from entering.

When a client does come in to a salon it is polite and good practice to make eye contact with them straightaway, even if you are busy with another client or taking a booking by

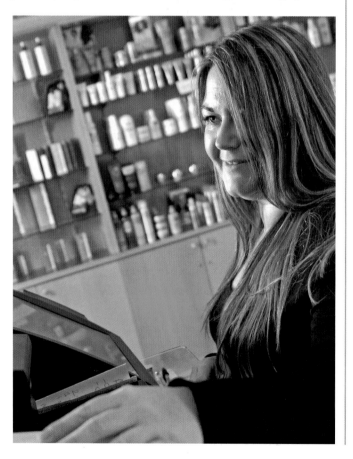

phone. This can relax a client, as they know that you have acknowledged them. Always smile, even when answering the telephone, as people can tell by the way you speak and the tone in your voice.

In most salons now refreshments and magazines are offered to clients, while they wait and as they are having their hair done. Make sure if you are offering refreshments that they are served well and not in dirty cups or with milk that has gone off. Good presentation means attention to detail, and is often noted by clients.

Offering to take a client's coat and belongings is also good practice, but do make sure that they are looked after and hung up or stored nicely so as not to damage them. When offering clients a seat in a waiting area or room, it is always a good idea to show them by pointing with the hand where to sit or even showing them through to the waiting area if it is not in the reception, as not doing so or being vague can confuse people and make them anxious.

Always mention a time scale for how long they will need to wait, but be approximate or they may complain if made to wait longer. Try to always run on time – clients do like this and hate having an appointment at 10am and being seen at 10.30am. It's not punctual and can be seen as bad manners, and they may feel rushed when your next client arrives. If you don't get the timings right from the start, you will be chasing your tail all day and neither you nor your clients will appreciate it.

Once seated, an assistant or the stylist should come and collect the client to take them to the workstation. This should be done before gowning a client, as you may need to assess their lifestyle and personality by their clothing. Make sure that you make contact with the client by shaking hands or introducing yourself, as this breaks the ice and makes the client feel comfortable.

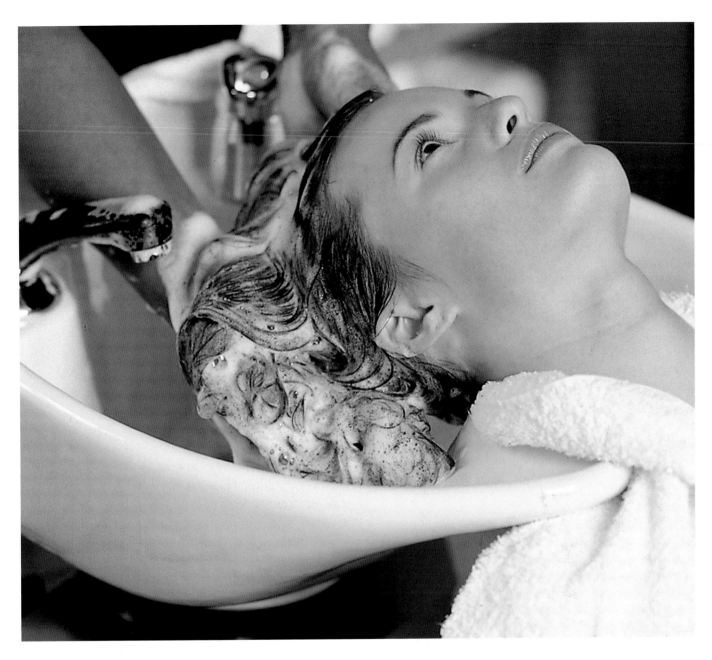

Once the client is in your chair, follow the consultation guide (see pages 26–33) and make sure you are polite and explain everything you are doing to reassure them. Be sure to advise clients of any hidden costs or extra time needed for the service up front.

Once the service is completed it is polite to go with the client to the reception or pay area, thank them, suggest that they book their next appointment there and then and ask if they are happy with the service they have had. Then hand them to the receptionist who should take care of returning their belongings, take their payment, book any further appointments, and check again that the client is happy.

If you want to go one step further and don't mind giving up the time, you could always give the client a call a week or so after their appointment and check that everything is OK. This is more for those clients whose hair you have changed drastically, or if they are using a product they are unfamiliar with or are new to the salon. Although some clients might see it as a little intrusive, you will be pleasantly surprised by how loyal clients can become with treatment like that. Just make sure that if you do it once and things change again, that you continue doing it.

# in the line of duty

Once you are qualified as a hairstylist, there are many different ways to use your skills and to gain experience and better your career. Many people who become hairdressers stay in salons for their whole career and are not aware that their skills can take them all over the globe and into many different angles of hairdressing.

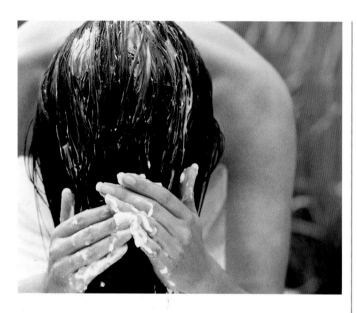

## Spa work

Many salons are now linked with spas or are even inside spas. This can alter the business entirely, as clients often come in for a full day of beauty pampering and then like to have their hair styled at the end of the day. In this line of work you find a lot of blow-drying, but regular clients can easily become loyal, full-service clients. You will learn more about body and beauty treatments and can often train in other areas such as manicures and pedicures.

## Health clubs

Another link has formed over the years with health clubs, where hair salons are located in the club's vicinity. These are often run as regular salons, but you get the added benefit of having club access.

## Mobile stylist

As a stylist you can of course go solo, without the premises. This is a great way of learning how to run your own business and building a clientele of your own. It can be hard work as you don't have any assistants, but can be rewarding if you have good, loyal clients.

## TV and film work

This angle of work is great experience if you like to try diverse hairstyling, as it requires many different techniques. Depending on what is being shot, you could be doing anything from 1940s hairstyles to aliens. It is a very different hairdressing job from regular salon work, and you may find that you need some stage makeup qualifications as well.

## Theatre

Often this work is similar to TV work and requires you to have knowledge of period hairstyles, different eras and stage makeup. It is very different to salon work as you don't have clients as such, and will probably do a lot of work on wigs instead of actual hair.

## Mortuary work

It may not be for everyone, but it's worth bearing in mind that hairdressers are employed by mortuaries to style dead people's hair. Although not to everyone's taste, it can be very well paid.

## Ships

Ship work is more or less like working in a salon, just at sea. However, you should expect to work very long hours, often for seven days a week. You will be expected to do a lot of formal styles for cocktail parties, a lot of blow-drying and not very much colour or cut work. It is often not well paid, but can pay well on commissions, and a huge advantage is that you can travel the world. Remember that you are at sea, which means that you are not covered by any country's rules for minimum wages or employees' rights.

# dealing with complaints

Unfortunately for all hairdressers, at some point or another, whether you are in training or fully qualified, you will have to deal with a complaint. It does not necessarily mean you have done the hair wrong or you have not cut or coloured it well – it may simply be that the client does not like it, or just a miscommunication, which is why it is important to do a thorough consultation. In a salon, complaints are normally referred to a manager who then will either deal with it themselves or pass it back to you – either way, you need to be prepared to deal with it.

Often in this situation a client may not want to come back to you, as they may be embarrassed or think you will be rude to them, but sometimes they will come back and it is how you deal with this that determines whether you can win the client back. It is very important to listen to your client first and really hear them, be sympathetic and try your hardest to win back their confidence in you before making suggestions or approaching how to fix the problem in question. Never get defensive or try to explain your actions – just focus on making it right.

Make a fuss of the client to make them feel even more welcome than before. Even thank them for coming and telling you that they were not happy. This may sound absurd, but it's better that a client comes back and complains than never comes back at all – at least you now have the opportunity to correct it.

If a client likes a service you have given them, they will go away feeling great and possibly tell one or two people before forgetting about you. However, if you make a mistake or they don't like what you've done, the whole world will know and they will talk about it for days to everyone they see. It really is to your advantage to thank them for coming back and talking to you about it.

An even better approach is to call the client a few days later or the day after and ask them if they are happy. This will eliminate the problem if they are not, and you can invite them to come back free of charge to correct whatever it is they do not like. If you don't call them, they may not come back to complain at all and just ask another salon to fix it – then you have lost your client.

Once somebody has complained it as also a good idea to

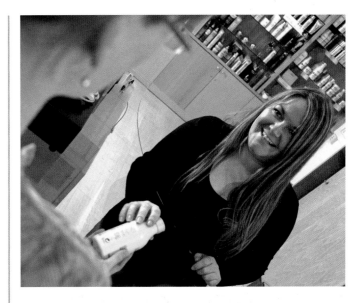

give them a small incentive to come back, such as a discount off their next appointment or a free treatment with their next cut. They may have come back, complained and had it corrected, but it does not mean you are out of the dog house!

If a client complains to a manager and refuses to have you redo their hair but will come back to another stylist, don't hide in the back room hoping to avoid them. It is courteous and professional to go to the client once they are in and settled, apologize and say how sorry you are that they did not like your work. Don't overdo it – just say your piece and then stay out of the way, but do be polite and possibly try to help the stylist who is redoing the hair. Offer the client refreshments or a magazine – this will show that you care and are being genuine.

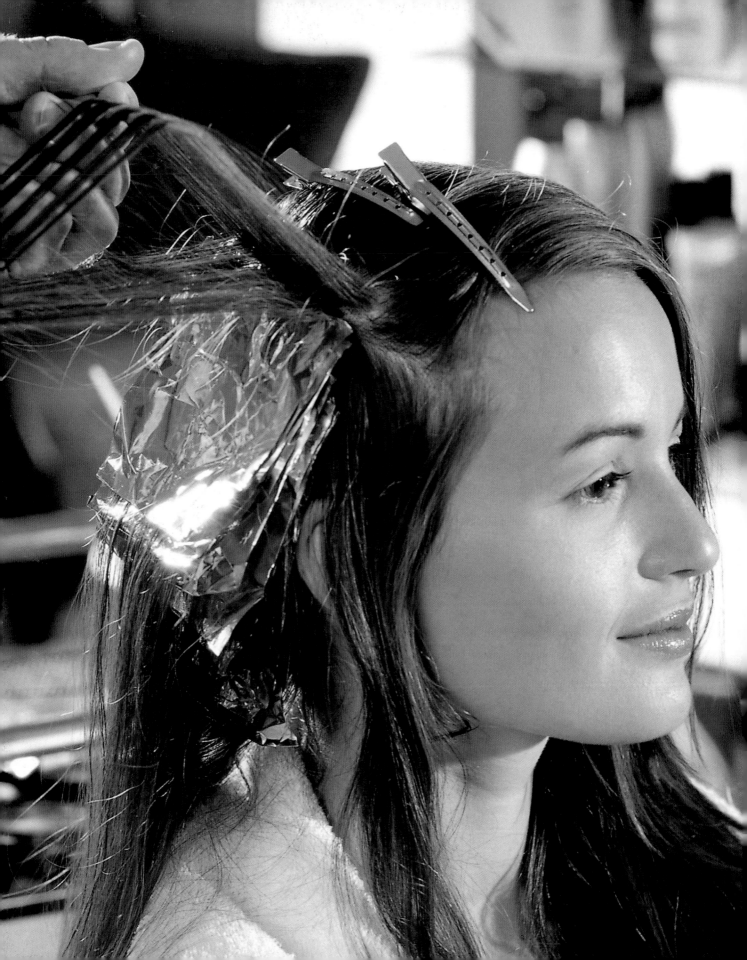

# 07 business checklist

# setting up a business

Running your own business can be very exciting: you are independent, with the freedom to choose what sort of salon you will have, how you will run it and who will work with you. But running a business requires huge self discipline, hard work, commitment, good decision-making, patience, drive and a lot of determination. There are also many things to consider when setting up a hairdressing business, and very little of it is as simple as cutting hair well.

There are several different ways of starting your business, but the most common are listed here:

## 1 Go mobile
Going mobile is a great way of starting a business without actually needing the premises to do it from. This would be a good starting point in hairdressing before eventually owning a salon, as you can build up your clientele and the only costs incurred are the equipment and petrol. Do bear in mind, though, that you would have to register with an accountant as you will be self-employed, which requires you to declare your earnings and pay your own tax, national insurance and other bills.

Going mobile can have its ups and downs. The pros are that you run your own books and appointment times, so if you don't want to do late nights or Sundays you don't have to. However, if you don't want to lose clients you may find that you will have to be very flexible. One of the cons is that if you chose to have a holiday for two weeks and don't have an employee to cover for you (which is unlikely, as not many mobile hairdressers have assistants), then be prepared to lose your clients as they may need you and have to go elsewhere.

## 2 Start from scratch
This will need lots of planning and can be risky. If you have worked in a salon or as a mobile hairdresser already and have a possible following clientele, this will help as it will bring in revenue straight away. If you are starting with no background in either of these areas, your business may take a while to build up both a reputation and a clientele, and it can cost you to employ a hairdresser who does have a clientele to follow them and bring in revenue.

This is not the best of ways to start unless you have done a lot of market research and have found an isolated, largely populated area that demands a hairdressing salon. As with any new business, it pays to do your homework.

## 3 Buy an existing business
In the hairdressing world, this is not always that easy. You may buy the salon and its equipment and inherit its good reputation, but there is still no guarantee that clients will stay and, after all, that's what you need the most as they pay the bills!

Salons that have been open for many years, where the proprietor is ready to retire, are often ripe for selling on, but be aware that these businesses are often old-fashioned and could need a lot of input to get them back on track. If a fairly new salon is for sale, find out why – it may not be doing well, and is possibly in a bad location. Check out the accounting books if you can, and investigate the earnings, profits and losses for previous years.

## 4 Buy into a franchise
There are many established franchises that operate all over the world, and you can buy the right to benefit from their name or brand. They often help with marketing, training and other operational support. They can be less risky than independent salons, but ultimately you have to run things by their rules and you can pay for it if you don't.

However, if you want to run under a well-established business name and want a very good guarantee of success, then this is for you. You will be well looked after and most businesses offer great opportunities in many areas, from fashion show work to photography, competitions and often travel.

# finance

When planning to start a business, you will often have to borrow money. For this, you will require a business plan, in which you must gather information and data about your planned business and how you intend to run it and make money.

You will need:
- ★ A plan of your facilities and services;
- ★ An idea of how much the services will cost;
- ★ Market research, e.g. questionnaires in the proposed area;
- ★ A list of equipment required and how much it costs;
- ★ Detailed analysis of the business and how it will run.

These are just a few of the things needed, but your money lender may request more and will often help you to put all the information together.

If you do not require financial support to open a business then you are lucky, but do remember that many of the above criteria still apply, and you would be well-advised to do your homework on both the business and the area in which you wish you open it. Money alone will not make a business flourish, so bear in mind that, along with your money, you will also need to invest a lot of hard work, time and devotion. It can take a long time to build up a good business, so do your research, put in the hours, hire the right staff and the rewards can be great.

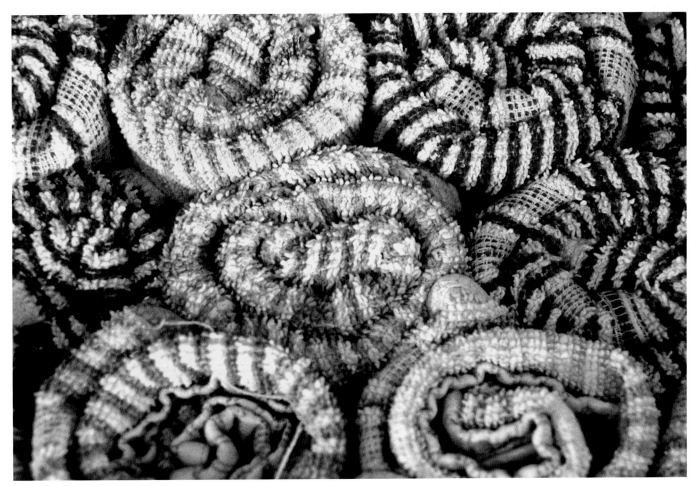

# legal obligations and costs

Once your business is almost up and running there are many issues you must be prepared for, and few of them will be as straightforward as cutting hair. A good manager needs to be able to deal with a lot of small but important details...

## Legal duties

★ Register as a business with the local authorities.
★ Register with Inland Revenue.
★ Register with an accountant who will deal with national insurance and tax issues (for a fee).
★ Salons often need to be assessed for health and hygiene – be sure to check this.
★ Salons also need to be assessed for fire risk and emergency exits, etc.
★ Equal rights rules must be adhered to when recruiting new staff.
★ Access for people with disabilities must be provided in many countries.
★ Employment laws and rules must be followed.

## Costs to bear in mind...

★ When the business is up and running, you will need to pay business rates.
★ Water rates, gas and electricity bills must be factored in to your plans.
★ Council tax for businesses must be paid.
★ You must be able to afford the equipment and products that are vital for your salon.
★ If you employ staff, you must be able to pay their wages.
★ You will need to look at insurance cover for your building, including health and safety issues, and it's worth looking into insurance protection for the business in case somebody wants to sue you.

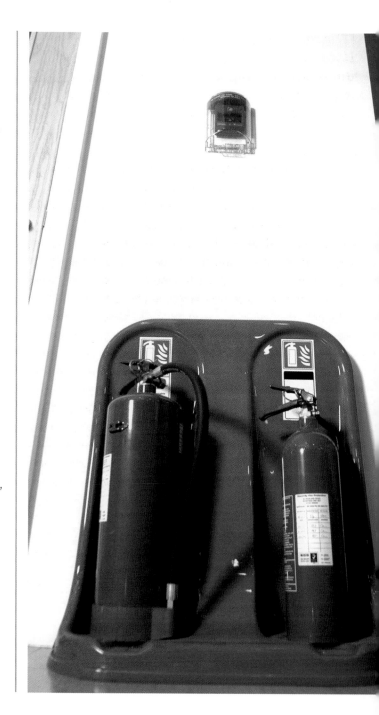

# staffing and equipment

If you lack experience in hairdressing, try if you can to hire an experienced hairstylist from a prestigious salon, who can not only help you find a team of professional and well-qualified hairdressers, but can also bring a large client following to your salon.

Employing the right staff is not easy, especially in the hairdressing industry, where stylists and assistants tend to move around a lot from job to job. One of the best ways to keep staff is to motivate them with incentives, and to encourage a fun, happy working environment.

## Equipment

When opening a salon, some larger hairdressing companies have deals that encourage you to use all their products and equipment. This can work to your advantage, as you don't have to buy it all at once and they either rent it to you or you pay for it in instalments. This can be helpful, as some of the larger hairdressing equipment can be very expensive and often you will have only one to two months to pay for products such as colours, styling products, etc. You can also order products regularly – even monthly – so you can avoid having to order in bulk and instead get just enough for your anticipated salon usage.

In the back of hair trade magazines, you can often find useful addresses for auctions or companies who sell equipment. Auctions can be great for new businesses, as they sometimes sell brand-new equipment from a salon that has closed, which you can get for a fraction of the price.

There are many items needed to equip a salon to the full, so creating a list of essential and non-essential items is a good idea to start you off.

**ESSENTIAL ITEMS**

- Reception desk
- Till, plus credit card machine
- Telephone
- Waiting seats
- Coat stand or rack
- Work stations
- Work station chairs
- Mirrors
- Backwashes
- Backwash chairs
- Heat machine, such as Climazon or Rollerball
- All hairdressing equipment (hairdryers, towels, rollers, brushes, combs, hood dryers, colour bowls, clips, nets, etc.)
- Many miscellaneous essentials such as stationery, robes, refreshment cups, soap for toilets and cleaning equipment, etc.

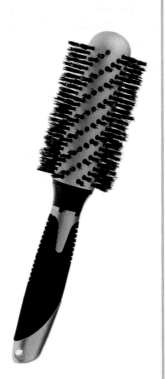

# location and marketing

Looking for the perfect location is crucial to how successful your business will be, and a great shop front can act as your own personal advert. Good window displays make a great first impression, but there are many other crucial factors.

Look for:
★ A good sized space
★ Parking
★ Easy access
★ Somewhere that people pass regularly
★ A shop front
★ A busy shopping area

It is also very important to note what is around your business – after all, it's no good having a fantastic salon in the middle of an industrial estate full of car mechanics and bathroom salesrooms. The best location for a thriving salon would be among clothes, fashion, makeup and anything to do with image.

The size and shape of your property is also important. If it's too small it would end up being cramped after you've fitted in all your equipment and staff, but if it's too big you have to fill it either with expensive gear or with clients, both of which can be tricky at first.

Parking is essential, as clients will expect a dedicated, free parking area. Not only can parking be difficult in the areas where salons usually are, but it can be hard to predict how long a client will be there. Parking with the premises can make all the difference to both clients and staff, but make sure you don't fill the car park with your staff's cars and leave no room for those precious clients who pay the bills.

Access is another important issue. Being upstairs is not a problem provided that you have a lift or escalator, but be aware that if access is not available to everyone, not only could you lose a loyal client who has a problem with stairs, but you could be in trouble with the law, which requires disabled access.

Once you have found your prime location, make sure to make your shop front presentable and eye-catching.

## TIPS FOR SUCCESS

### 1 Choose the right location
Find a great location with lots of people around, unless you have a great clientele already that will follow you anywhere.

### 2 Offer a clean and safe working environment
Make sure your new business environment is clean and safe to work in for you and all your staff, and that it stays that way.

### 3 Hire the right qualified staff
Employ people who you think will suit your business and its image and will work well for you and as a team. Make sure they hold good qualifications and even do a trade test on them first, before hiring.

### 4 Offer great service
Try to offer other services such as manicures and possibly even beauty treatments that enhance your business. If not, make sure that the services you do offer are of the highest standard and cover a large range of treatments, so that none of your clients need to go elsewhere.

### 5 Keep your clients satisfied
A salon's best marketing tool is word of mouth, and once one client has had a great experience with you, they will often spread the word to friends, relatives and colleagues. This can multiply your clients over time. Always look after your client's needs, use their feedback to establish how you are doing, and always keep them satisfied.

# the salon

Once you have found your location, you need to plan the space. Think about the flow of the room – for instance, when the clients first enter the salon, you need a reception then a waiting area, possibly with a cloakroom, then you need to have stations for the main work area and backwashes. You also need a staffroom, a place to make coffee and tea and toilet facilities, and the better this is planned, the better the flow of the salon will be.

After deciding on where things will go, you need to decide on the look: will it be neutral wood, black and white, Mediterranean-looking, etc. Many salon groups have a corporate look which solves the problem, but if you are independent then you need to choose carefully. What sort of clients are you hoping to attract? Going too modern can be off-putting for older clients, but too fusty and you will not attract a younger, potentially more fashionable clientele. Looks can also date very quickly, so keep it simple and classy and use accessories that can be updated cheaply when necessary.

Many companies that stock and set up salons will have lots of ideas for you and can sometimes help with floorplans, too. If you know a good joiner, there have been many salons that have started out with handmade stations and reception areas – this can save you money and give a unique look, and once the money starts coming in you can redo it according to budget.

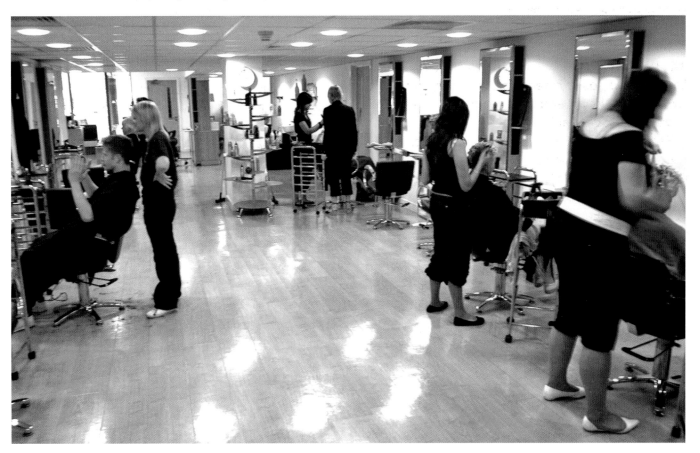

# glossary

**ammonium thioglycollate** The main ingredient used in perm lotion.
**analysis** The process of working out what chemicals are already on the hair.
**ash** A cool hair colour.

**base colour** Black/brown/blonde of all shades.
**brick** A sectioning and winding technique for perms.
**brittle** Very dry and rough feeling.

**channel cutting** Cutting hair while sliding the scissors over the top.
**chip cutting** Cutting small, uneven amounts in V-shapes.
**club cutting** Cutting straight into the hair to create one steady weight line.
**consultation** To talk to a client to find out what they want.
**cortex** The inner core of hair.
**cuticle** The outer sheath of hair.

**dandruff** Dead skin cells that are shed from the scalp.
**density** Amount of hair.
**directional** Hair wound in a certain direction. Also a sectioning pattern for perms.
**disulphide bond** A bond in the hair's structure that is altered when perming hair.

**elasticity** The hair's ability to stretch without breaking and then return to its original shape.

**floodlight** A colouring technique.

**henna** A vegetable dye made from the leaves and stems of a henna plant. Gives hair a reddish colour.
**highlights** The subtle lifting of colour in specific sections of hair.
**hydrogen peroxide** The main ingredient in perm neutralizer.

**ICC** International Colour Code.

**lowlights** The subtle darkening of colour in specific sections of hair.

**manufacturer's instructions** Leaflet supplied by a maker of a product indicating how and how not to use it.
**melanin** and **pheomelanin** The pigments which naturally colour the hair and skin.
**molton browner** A flexible, bendy roller.

**neutralize** To reset or counteract a perming chemical.
**nine section** Hair divided into nine sections, used either for perming or colouring.

**oxidant** or **peroxide** Hydrogen peroxide liquid – the main ingredient in perm neutralizer.

**paddle brush** Flat, wide brush used to dry hair straight.
**paint-on** A colouring technique.
**permanent colour** Colour that either grows out or is cut out.
**personalizing** To make a cut unique to and/or suitable for the client.
**piggy back** A winding technique for perms.
**porosity** The hair's ability to absorb moisture.
**primary colour** The three main colours that all other colours are derived from.

**quasi colour** A colour that is neither semi-permanent nor permanent.

**reconstructing** To rebuild hair and make it stronger.
**relaxer** The same process as perming that straightens hair instead.

**retail** To sell products.

**sebum** Natural oils in the skin and scalp that lubricate and protect.
**secondary colours** Colours made of two primary colours.
**sectioning** or **section** To divide the hair into areas prior to cutting or colouring.
**semi-permanent colour** Colour that lasts around 6–8 washes.
**sensitized hair** Internally damaged hair.
**shoe-shine** A colouring technique.
**skin test** A test done to check for adverse reactions to colour.
**slicing** A cutting technique that removes weight and bulk.
**smudge** A colouring technique.
**snapper brush** Two brushes facing each other attached by a spring. Used for drying hair straight.

**tail comb** Comb with a plastic comb at one end and a metal or plastic prong at the other.
**texture** The thickness of hair.
**thermal** Anything to do with heat application.
**thinning** Cutting small pieces of hair to a shorter length to reduce overall bulk and heaviness.
**tones** Colours that enhance and change natural colours.

**undercoat** Natural tones under the hair colour.

**virgin hair** Hair with no chemical alterations ever done to it.
**visuals** Consultation aids that help you and a client agree on what is wanted. Can be photos, magazines, colour charts, etc.

**warm** Yellow, red or orange based undertones in hair, skin, or makeup.

# index

# acknowledgements

All photography is by Paul West with the exception of the photographs listed below. These are by Micky Hoyle for New Holland Image Library.

Page 11
Page 24–27
Page 29–36
Page 37 (right)
Page 38–39
Page 45
Page 80 (right)
Page 142
Page 147–148
Page 150
Page 155

New Holland Publishers would like to thank the following:

Arena Hair & Beauty, Kingston
Vanessa Green
Anna Breugem
Jo Partrick
Alice Royston-Lee
Rosie Watson
Penny Brown